Endodontology
at a Glance

Endodontology
at a Glance

Alix Davies

BDS (Hons), MFDS, MJDF, MClinDent, MEndo
Specialist in Endodontics/Clinical Tutor
King's College London Dental Institute
& Specialist Practice, London, UK

Federico Foschi

BDS, MSc, PhD, FDS, FHEA
Consultant/Honorary Senior Lecturer in
Endodontics
King's College London Dental Institute
& Specialist Practice, London, UK

Shanon Patel

BDS, MSc, MClinDent, MRD, PhD, FDS, FHEA
Consultant/Honorary Reader in Endodontics
King's College London Dental Institute
& Specialist Practice, London, UK

WILEY Blackwell

The right of Alix Davies, Federico Foschi and Shanon Patel to be identified as the authors of the material in this work has been asserted in accordance with law.

Registered Offices
John Wiley & Sons, Inc., 111 River Street, Hoboken, NJ 07030, USA
John Wiley & Sons Ltd, The Atrium, Southern Gate, Chichester,
West Sussex, PO19 8SQ, UK

Editorial Office
9600 Garsington Road, Oxford, OX4 2DQ, UK

For details of our global editorial offices, customer services, and more information about Wiley products visit us at www.wiley.com.

Wiley also publishes its books in a variety of electronic formats and by print-on-demand. Some content that appears in standard print versions of this book may not be available in other formats.

Limit of Liability/Disclaimer of Warranty
The contents of this work are intended to further general scientific research, understanding, and discussion only and are not intended and should not be relied upon as recommending or promoting scientific method, diagnosis, or treatment by physicians for any particular patient. In view of ongoing research, equipment modifications, changes in governmental regulations, and the constant flow of information relating to the use of medicines, equipment, and devices, the reader is urged to review and evaluate the information provided in the package insert or instructions for each medicine, equipment, or device for, among other things, any changes in the instructions or indication of usage and for added warnings and precautions. While the publisher and authors have used their best efforts in preparing this work, they make no representations or warranties with respect to the accuracy or completeness of the contents of this work and specifically disclaim all warranties, including without limitation any implied warranties of merchantability or fitness for a particular purpose. No warranty may be created or extended by sales representatives, written sales materials or promotional statements for this work. The fact that an organization, website, or product is referred to in this work as a citation and/or potential source of further information does not mean that the publisher and authors endorse the information or services the organization, website, or product may provide or recommendations it may make. This work is sold with the understanding that the publisher is not engaged in rendering professional services. The advice and strategies contained herein may not be suitable for your situation. You should consult with a specialist where appropriate. Further, readers should be aware that websites listed in this work may have changed or disappeared between when this work was written and when it is read. Neither the publisher nor authors shall be liable for any loss of profit or any other commercial damages, including but not limited to special, incidental, consequential, or other damages.

Library of Congress Cataloging-in-Publication Data

Names: Davies, Alix, author. | Foschi, Federico, author. | Patel, Shanon, author.
Title: Endodontology at a glance / Alix Davies, Federico Foschi, Shanon Patel.
Description: Hoboken, NJ : Wiley-Blackwell, 2018. | Series: At a glance series |
   Includes index. |
Identifiers: LCCN 2018034896 (print) | LCCN 2018035389 (ebook) | ISBN
   9781118994719 (Adobe PDF) | ISBN 9781118994726 (ePub) | ISBN 9781118994702 (pbk.)
Subjects: | MESH: Dental Pulp Diseases—diagnosis | Dental Pulp
   Diseases—therapy | Root Canal Therapy | Endodontics—methods | Handbooks
Classification: LCC RK351 (ebook) | LCC RK351 (print) | NLM WU 49 | DDC
   617.6/342—dc23
LC record available at https://lccn.loc.gov/2018034896

Cover image: © Shanon Patel
Cover design by Wiley

Set in Minion Pro 9.5/11.5 by Aptara
Printed and bound in Singapore by Markono Print Media Pte Ltd

10 9 8 7 6 5 4 3 2 1

Dedications

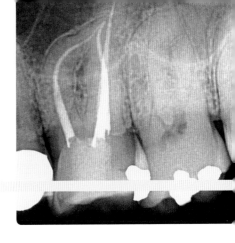

Alix dedicates this book to her husband Paul, her children James and Isobel, and her parents Leigh and John.

Federico dedicates the book to Martina, Alessandro and Arianna.

Shanon dedicates the book to Almas, Genie and Zarina.

Contents

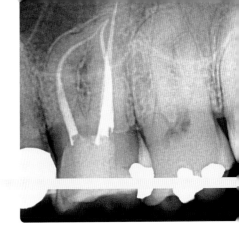

About the companion website

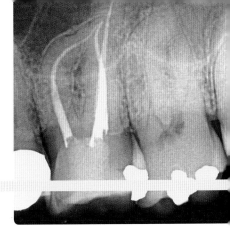

Don't forget to visit the companion website for this book:

www.wiley.com/go/davies/endodontology

There you will find valuable material designed to enhance your learning:

* Interactive multiple choice questions

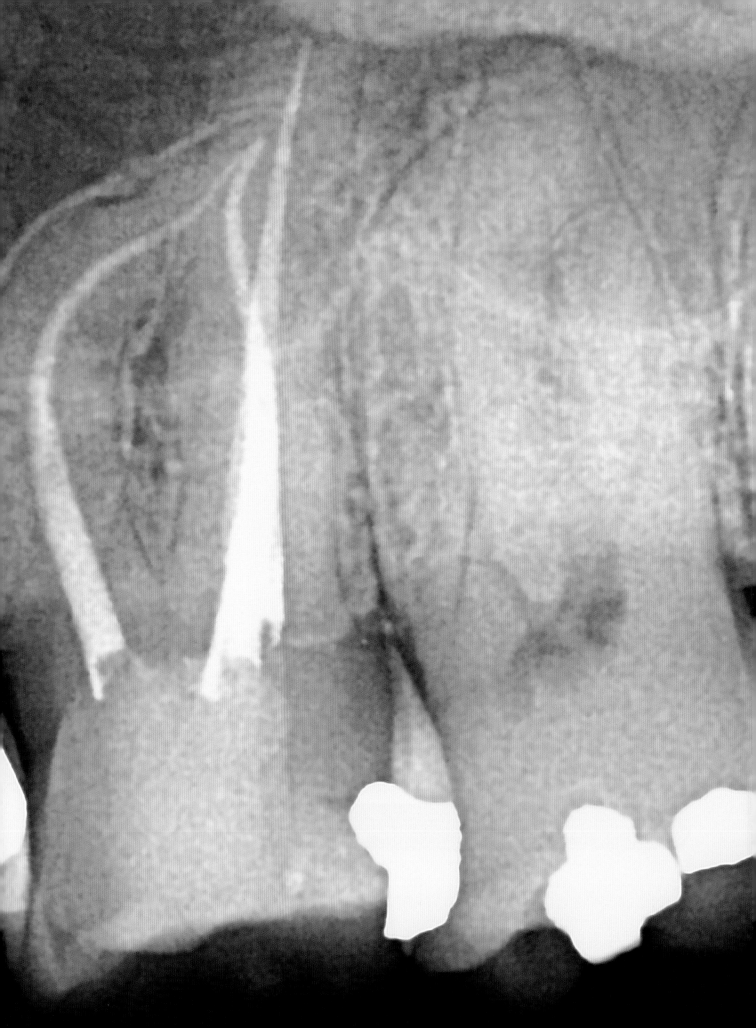

Disease processes in endodontology

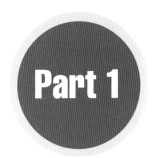

Part 1

Chapters

The causes and sequelae of endodontic disease

Figure 1.1 Section of tooth showing a carious lesion. Between this and the pulp, tertiary dentine deposition and intratubular sclerosis can be seen.
Source: Courtesy of Ahmed Ali.

Figure 1.2 Periapical radiograph of the UL2 showing radiographic signs of chronic apical periodontitis associated with an infected necrotic pulp.

Figure 1.3 Periapical radiograph of the LR6 showing radiographic signs of chronic apical periodontitis associated with an existing root filling.

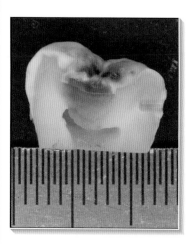

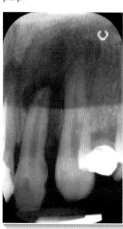

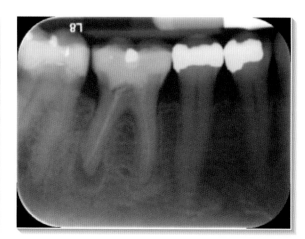

Table 1.1 The roles of acute inflammatory mediators.

Mediator	Source	Role
Histamine	Mast cells, basophils	Vasodilatation, increased permeability
Prostaglandins	Mast cells, leucocytes	Vasodilatation
Leukotrienes	Mast cells, leucocytes	Increased permeability, leucocyte chemotaxis and adhesion
Platelet activating factor	Mast cells, leucocytes	Vasodilatation, increased permeability
Cytokines (IL1, TNF)	Mast cells, macrophages	Endothelial activation, fibroblast proliferation, neutrophil chemotaxis
Nitric oxide	Macrophages, endothelium	Vasodilatation
Complement	Plasma	Leucocyte chemotaxis and activation
Kinins	Plasma	Vasodilatation, increased permeability
Fibrinogen	Plasma	Chemotaxis and migration of neutrophils

Pulpitis is the inflammation of the pulp, whereas apical periodontitis is the inflammation of the tissues surrounding the apex of the tooth, including the periodontal ligament and the alveolar bone. Inflammation can be acute or chronic.

Acute inflammation

Acute inflammation is characterised by:
- Redness
- Heat
- Swelling
- Pain
- Loss of function.

The redness and heat produced in an area of acute inflammation are the results of vessel dilatation and increased blood flow to that area. Swelling is caused by the accumulation of tissue exudates which contain neutrophils and inflammatory mediators (Table 1.1). The exudate aims to dilute the toxins whilst the neutrophils ingest the pathogens by phagocytosis. Pain is felt because of the swelling exerting pressure on nerve endings. Certain chemical mediators can also stimulate pain receptors. Swelling and pain can result in loss of function of the inflamed area.

Chronic inflammation

Acute inflammation can be reversible by removal of the damaging stimulus. However, if it persists, chronic inflammation ensues. Chronic inflammation is the result of a balance between continued tissue damage and attempts by the host to eradicate the disease to produce some tissue repair. Macrophages are among the main effector cells in chronic inflammation. They secrete various inflammatory mediators and have a role in phagocytosis and antigen presentation. Lymphocytes additionally recognise foreign antigens by binding to them before proliferating to mount an immune response by cell-mediated immunity (T lymphocytes) or by humoral immunity (B lymphocytes). Symptoms are usually limited at the chronic inflammation stage.

Causes of apical periodontitis

Apical periodontitis is caused by bacterial infection of the pulp. In a healthy tooth, the pulp dentine complex is protected from oral microorganisms by the overlying enamel and cementum. However, these layers can be damaged by caries, cracks or fractures, tooth wear, restorative procedures or periodontal procedures to produce portals of entry for microorganisms.

As bacteria penetrate into dentine, they release toxins that pass through the dentine tubules. The pulp responds to this by producing a layer of tertiary dentine as an additional protective layer. Increased intratubular mineral deposition may also reduce the permeability of the dentine (Figure 1.1). However, once the microorganisms penetrate into the inner dentine layers, the toxins they produce cause significant pulpal inflammation. If no treatment is provided, the bacteria eventually invade and colonise the pulp. The pulp is encased in a hard dentine shell and can therefore not expand to accommodate large amounts of fluid exudate. It also lacks sufficient collateral circulation. These factors limit the ability of the pulp to respond effectively to the insult. Pulpal inflammation can initially be reversible, with removal of the irritants resulting in resolution of the inflammation. However, as the immune challenge increases, the pulpal damage will advance beyond repair, resulting in irreversible inflammation and progressive pulpal necrosis.

Restorative procedures additionally may 'push' a tooth with pre-existing pulpal inflammation to irreversible pulpitis. This occurs by overheating, desiccation or chemical irritation to the dentino-pulp complex. If rubber dam is not used, or poor fitting temporary restorations are placed, microleakage can also occur. The risk of permanent damage is higher when the restorative work is close to the pulp and the dentine is permeable.

A root canal with a necrotic pulp is the ideal environment for bacterial colonisation as it provides a warm, moist, nutritious and anaerobic environment. The reduced presence of oxygen can also select aggressive anaerobic pathogens. The microorganisms are protected from the host defences as there is no blood circulation in the necrotic tissue. They derive their nutrients from the necrotic pulp tissue, periradicular tissue fluids, saliva and metabolic by-products of other bacterial species.

Over time, the bacteria progress apically down the root canal. Leakage of toxins and metabolic by-products through the apical foramen also stimulates the inflammatory response in the periapical tissues. Inflammatory mediators are released that stimulate osteoclast differentiation. This results in apical bone resorption and production of an apical lesion surrounded by chronic inflammatory cells. This stage of the disease is described as chronic apical periodontitis associated with an infected necrotic tooth (Figure 1.2).

The aim of root canal treatment is to reduce the bacterial load and seal the canals to prevent further ingress of bacteria. However, chronic inflammation can persist if inadequate disinfection is performed, with microorganisms remaining at levels sufficient to stimulate an inflammatory response. If the root canal system and coronal aspect of the tooth are not adequately sealed after root canal treatment, bacteria can re-enter and cause recurrence of the apical inflammation. It can be difficult to identify if the cause of the inflammation is persistence of, or re-entry of bacteria (or both). This stage of the disease is described as chronic apical periodontitis associated with an infected root-filled tooth (Figure 1.3).

Bacteria can egress through the apical foramen and, in some cases, cause suppuration that presents as an acute apical abscess or a chronic sinus tract.

Microbiology of apical periodontitis

Figure 2.1 Stages in biofilm development.

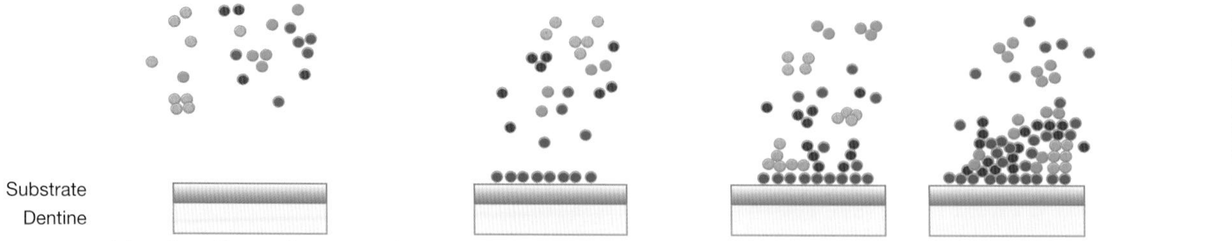

Substrate
Dentine

Adsorption of inorganic and organic molecules to the root canal wall to produce a conditioning layer → Attachment of planktonic microorganisms to produce a monolayer → Secondary colonisers are attracted to the monolayer, increasing its thickness and complexity

Table 2.1 Advantages and disadvantages of culturing and molecular technology.

Method of microorganism detection	Advantages	Disadvantages
Culturing	• Broad range allowing for growth of unanticipated species • Relative quantities of microorganisms can be ascertained • Widely available • Pathogenicity and bacterial sensitivities can be performed	• A large number of microorganisms are uncultivatable • Some strains are ambiguous and not identifiable • Samples require immediate processing • Cultivation can be time consuming and costly • Low sensitivitiy
Molecular technology	• High sensitivity and specificity • Can detect cultivatable and non-cultivatable microorganisms • Rapid technique • Species can be detected directly from the clinical sample • Samples can be frozen for later analysis • Can detect dead microorganisms	• Information is mostly qualitative only, limited information about relative quantities • Assays can only detect a few species at a time • Usually performed to search for target species • Very expensive

Table 2.2 Comparison between primary and persistent infection of the root canals.

Microbiological feature	Primary apical periodontitis	Persistent apical periodontitis
Numbers of bacteria per root canal	1000 to 100 000 000	1000 to 10 000 000
Number of species per canal	10 to 20	1 to 5 (10 to 20 in poorly treated canals)
Prevalent bacterial species (gram negative)	*Fusobacterium, Porphyromonas, Prevotella, Treponema, Campylobacter, Veillonella*	*Fusobacterium, Prevotella, Camplylobacter*
Prevalent bacterial species (gram positive)	*Peptostreptococcus, Actinomyces, Eubacterium*	*Peptostreptococcus, Proprionibacterium, Lactobacillae, Enterococcus faecalis, Actinomyces*
Presence of fungi	Fungi less likely to be present	Fungi more likely to be present
Presence of *Enterococcus faecalis* in canals	Low prevalence	Very high prevalence

Endodontology at a Glance. First Edition. Alix Davies, Federico Foschi and Shanon Patel. © 2019 John Wiley & Sons, Ltd. Published 2019 by John Wiley & Sons, Ltd.
Companion website: www.wiley.com/go/davies/endodontology

Which methods of sampling are used for bacterial detection?

Apical periodontitis is caused by the presence of microorganisms and their toxins in the root canals causing progressive inflammation and necrosis of the pulp, followed by inflammation of the periapical tissues. Root canal treatment aims to reduce the microbial load to a level that permits the body to amount an effective immune response and promote healing. It has therefore been considered important to ascertain which microorganisms are present in the root canals of teeth with apical periodontitis to understand how the disease progresses, as well as how to manage it.

Methods for isolation and detection of endodontic microorganisms fall into culturing and molecular technology (Table 2.1). For each, a sample must be taken from the root canal. This is normally performed with paper points. This will normally only allow sampling of microorganisms that are present in the main canal lumen. Files assist in collecting 'scrapings' from the canal walls. Collection of bacteria from dentine tubules and isthmuses is very difficult.

Culturing

The sample is transported in a medium that preserves viability whilst not enhancing growth. The microbes are then distributed onto agar media or cultured in broths under aerobic or anaerobic conditions. Species can then be identified by assessing features including colony and cellular morphology, tolerance to oxygen, gram staining and metabolic end-product analysis. Other tests that can be performed on the microorganisms include susceptibility to certain antibiotics, oxygen tolerance and cell wall profile.

Molecular technology

Molecular technology enables identification of microorganisms without the need for culturing. It can more reliably identify bacteria, including those strains that show ambiguous phenotypes. Fungi can be identified by their 18S RNA gene. The clinical sample is solubilised, DNA extracted and specific nucleic acid probes (primers) are added that are complementary to the target species being investigated. If the target species is present, hybridisation will occur. The polymerase chain reaction will then amplify the DNA to a level at which it can be detected. If the target species are absent in the sample, no hybridisation will occur and no DNA will be amplified. Electrophoresis and fluorescent *in situ* hybridisation can be used to assist with separation and visual identification of the strains present.

Which bacteria are responsible for causing apical periodontitis?

The culturing and molecular biology techniques have revealed the presence of more than 400 microorganisms. Different bacteria dominate the canals in primary and persistent cases of apical periodontitis (Table 2.2).

Where do the bacteria reside in the root canal system?

Bacteria occur in the main canal as well as in accessory canals, isthmuses and deltas in the following habitats:

1 The lumen in planktonic form
2 The canals walls as part of a biofilm
3 The dentinal tubules.

A biofilm is a bacterial population that is embedded in a polysaccharide matrix and adheres to surfaces of solid–liquid interfaces (Figure 2.1). Biofilms are present in the root canal system and occasionally are extraradicular. The biofilm is advantageous to the microorganism in the following ways:

- **Broader habitat range for growth:** early colonisers alter the local environment and can increase nutrient availability and remove waste products. This enables other bacterial species that would not have survived alone to attach to, and form part of the biofilm.
- **Increased metabolic diversity and efficiency:** bacteria cohabiting in biofilms develop food webs whereby the metabolic by-products from one species become the main food source for another. Interactions between different species also allow more effective breakdown and utilisation of host-derived substrates compared with the actions of a single species alone.
- **Protection from the host defences:** the extracellular polysaccharide resists phagocytosis from the host inflammatory cells. In addition, various species can produce different enzymes to neutralise the host inflammatory mediators and also inactivate antibacterial solutions that can be used to remove them during root canal treatment. Antibiotics usually require a level of bacterial activity to be effective. However, bacteria in biofilms often grow more slowly and are at the stationary phase of growth for longer. This can result in enhanced antibiotic resistance.
- **Genetic exchange:** methods such as conjugation, transformation and transduction enable dissemination of virulence and antibiotic resistance genes within bacterial species of the biofilm.
- **Enhances pathogenicity:** bacteria which individually have a low virulence can still have a role in causing disease when they partake in a biofilm. Their role can be to assist the survival of more virulent bacteria by improving adherence of the biofilm to host surfaces, obtaining nutrients from the host and evading host defences.

How does the knowledge of the bacterial species and habitats influence endodontic treatment?

The complexity of intracanal infection requires treatment with a broad spectrum antibacterial such as sodium hypochlorite. Antimicrobial agents are far less effective at destroying bacteria in biofilms than planktonic bacteria. They will therefore need to be used in greater concentrations, or employed with techniques such as ultrasonic irrigation to disrupt the biofilms. Whilst microorganisms present in the main root canal can be directly accessed and ideally eliminated by instrumentation and irrigation, those microbes that are located in lateral canals and dentine tubules are more difficult to reach and can require other therapeutic strategies to eliminate them (see Chapter 12).

3 Resorption

Figure 3.1 Classification of root resorption.

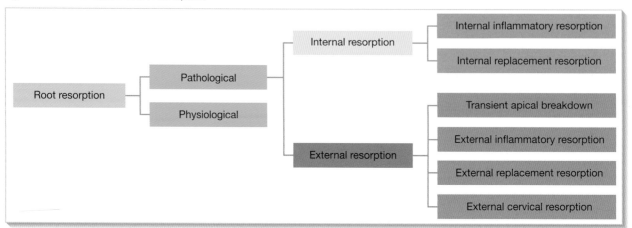

Root resorption
- Pathological
  - Internal resorption
    - Internal inflammatory resorption
    - Internal replacement resorption
  - External resorption
    - Transient apical breakdown
    - External inflammatory resorption
    - External replacement resorption
    - External cervical resorption
- Physiological

Figure 3.2 Diagrams showing the various ways resorptive lesions present: (a) internal inflammatory resorption, (b) external inflammatory resorption, and (c) external cervical resorption.

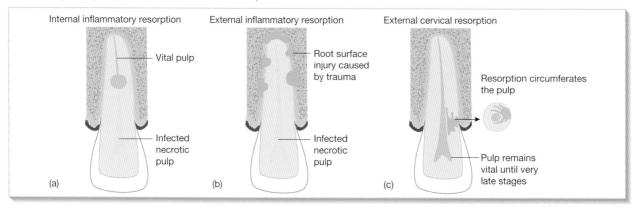

Internal inflammatory resorption
- Vital pulp
- Infected necrotic pulp
(a)

External inflammatory resorption
- Root surface injury caused by trauma
- Infected necrotic pulp
(b)

External cervical resorption
- Resorption circumferates the pulp
- Pulp remains vital until very late stages
(c)

Table 3.1 Predisposing factors and clinical features of root resorption.

| | Internal root resorption | | External root resorption | | |
	Inflammatory	Replacement	Inflammatory	Replacement	Cervical
Possible predisposing factors	• Trauma • Caries • Orthodontic treatment • Cracked teeth • Calcium hydroxide procedures on vital teeth • Periodontal infections • Heat generation during restorative procedures on vital teeth		• Trauma • Orthodontic treatment • Periodontal infections		• Trauma • Orthodontic procedures • Intracoronal bleaching • Surgical procedures • Periodontal therapy • Bruxism • Developmental defects
Clinical features	• Vital in early stages, negative in advanced cases • Usually asymptomatic • Pinkish hue (rare)		• Negative response to vitality tests • Usually asymptomatic	• Infraoccluded • Tooth immobile • High pitched percussive tone	• Located at the cervical margin • Pink spot may be noted by the patient/clinician • Profuse bleeding when probed • Sharp edges around the resorption cavity
Radiographical features	• Uniform enlargement of the root canal • Outline of the root canal is distorted • Usually no accompanying bone resorption	• Radiolucent (inflammatory) • Mottled (replacement)	• Chance radiological finding • Root canal outline is visible and intact	• Radiolucent (inflammatory) • Radiopaque (replacement)	• Chance radiological finding • Radiolucent (early), mottled (advanced) lesions • The root canal walls are visible and intact

Endodontology at a Glance. First Edition. Alix Davies, Federico Foschi and Shanon Patel. © 2019 John Wiley & Sons, Ltd. Published 2019 by John Wiley & Sons, Ltd.
Companion website: www.wiley.com/go/davies/endodontology

Root resorption is the loss of dental hard tissues as a result of clastic action. Physiological (primary dentition) root resorption allows permanent successors to erupt. However, any resorption of permanent teeth is pathological.

Pathological resorption may be internal or external, depending on the location of the resorptive lesion (Figure 3.1).

Internal root resorption

Internal inflammatory and internal replacement resorption

Pathogenesis and aetiology

The odontoblast/predentine layers of the pulpo-dentine complex must be damaged resulting in exposure of mineralised dentine. The aetiology is poorly understood (Table 3.1).

When coronal pulp tissue is inflamed because of bacterial ingress, inflammatory mediators stimulate recruitment of odontoclasts from the more apical pulpal blood supply. These bind to and resorb mineralised tissue. Internal resorption will only progress with bacterial stimulation and a vital blood supply to provide nutrients.

Internal replacement resorption occurs when hard tissue resembling bone (osteoid) or cementum is deposited (reparative phase) within the resorptive cavity.

Clinical and radiographic findings

• Internal inflammatory resorption can present with symptoms and/or signs of pulpal and/or periapical disease (Table 3.1).
• May be an incidental (asymptomatic) finding on radiography.

Specific management considerations

• A cone beam computed tomography (CBCT) scan is recommended in teeth considered restorable to determine the nature and extent of the resorptive defect.
• Endodontic treatment is recommended in restorable cases.
• An interappointment calcium hydroxide medicament can be placed to exert an antibacterial effect on tissue inaccessible to instrumentation.
• Obturate with thermoplasticised gutta percha to ensure that the complex root canal system is encompassed.
• Microsurgery is additionally required if there is an existing perforation.

External root resorption

Transient apical breakdown

Pathogenesis and aetiology

Rare radiological phenomenon caused by the localised transient inflammatory response (i.e. repair) associated with removal of necrotic tissue from the apices of traumatized teeth.

Clinical and radiographic findings

• Discoloration;
• A small periapical radiolucency develops soon after the initial dental trauma, but usually resolves (i.e. repair) within 3 months of the injury;
• There may initially be a negative response to pulp testing;
• Usually resolves within 12 months.

External inflammatory resorption

Pathogenesis and aetiology

Injury to the tooth by various aetiological factors (Table 3.1) can damage the cementum externally, exposing the underlying mineralised dentine.

The injury also results in pulpal necrosis and subsequent bacterial infection. Bacterial toxins pass through the dentine tubules, inducing an inflammatory response on the external aspect of the root. Osteoclasts migrate to the area and bind to and resorb the damaged exposed (mineralised) dentine.

Clinical and radiographic findings

• Signs and symptoms of pulpal and/or periapical disease or be asymptomatic.
• The radiograph will show a loss of tooth structure and radiolucencies in the adjacent bone. The root canal outline is seen through the radiographic defect.
• Early to moderate signs of external inflammatory resorption, especially on the labial or lingual aspects of the tooth, can be missed because of the two-dimensional nature of radiographs.

Management

• Root canal treatment with inter-appointment calcium hydroxide dressing.
• Microsurgery is sometimes required if a perforation is present.

External replacement resorption

The root becomes mistakenly incorporated into the remodelling process of the alveolar bone.

Pathogenesis and aetiology

In severe intrusion or avulsion injuries where the PDL is crushed and desiccated.

The irreversibly damaged periodontal ligament and adjacent root are resorbed by osteoclasts and 'replaced' with bone produced by osteoblasts from the adjacent alveolar bone. The pulp tissue does not have a role in the progression of the resorption.

Clinical findings

• High pitched metallic sound to percussion and no mobility in advanced cases.
• There may be no other signs of endo/perio disease.
• Radiologically resorption will only be detected on the proximal surfaces, where portions of the root are replaced with bone.

Management

No effective treatment and the tooth will eventually be lost.

External cervical resorption (ECR)

Pathogenesis and aetiology

Damage to cementum at the cervical margin below the epithelial attachment exposes mineralised dentine to osteoclasts which resorb the underlying dentine. Bone-like material may be deposited in an attempt to repair the resorbed dentine. The pulp has no role in stimulating ECR. There is no firm evidence for any of these aetiological factors (Table 3.1).

Diagnosis

• Usually asymptomatic and will respond to vitality testing, as the pulp is not involved until the advanced stages (Table 3.1).
• Defect usually identified by probing or scaling.
  • It will have sharp borders and a hard scratchy base.
  • Profuse bleeding on probing.
• Proximal resorptive lesions can be noticed as chance radiographic findings. There is no classic radiographic appearance.
  • Radiolucent (early)-radiopaque/mottled (advanced). Root canal will be intact.

Management

Treatment depends on the location, restorability and accessibility. CBCT is advisable to assess the nature of ECR prior to management. Treatment options include:
• external repair +/− endodontic treatment
• internal repair and root canal treatment,
• intentional replantation,
• periodic review (untreatable teeth),
• extraction (untreatable teeth).

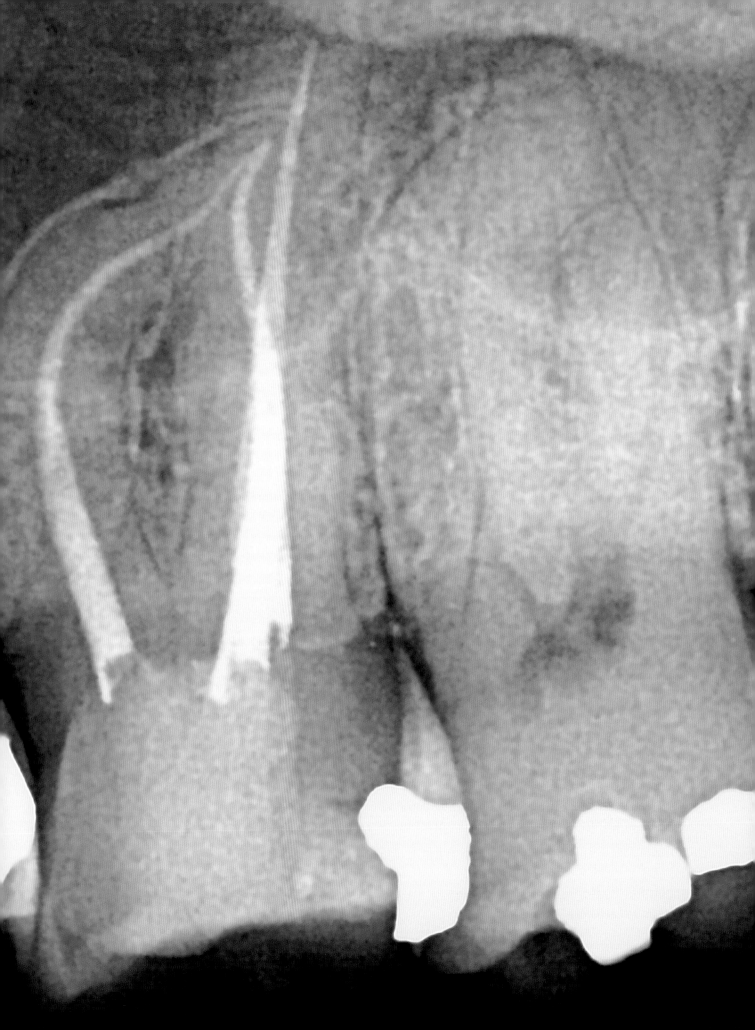

Diagnosis

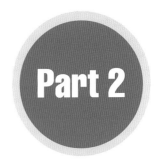

Part 2

Chapters

4 History taking

Table 4.1 Advantages and disadvantages of open and closed questioning.

	Open questions	**Closed questions**
Advantages	• Patient feels more involved • Patient can express all their concerns, some of these may be missed if just closed questions are asked • The way in which the patient answers the questions will give the dentist some insight into the type of patient they are managing. They can tailor their explanations and responses more appropriately	• Useful to gain additional information from patients who will not willingly divulge it • Allows the dentist to clarify information • Relevant information can be gathered more quickly
Disadvantages	• The consultation can be longer • The patient can provide information that is not relevant	• The clinician may not gain all the facts from the patient • The patient may feel rushed • Leading questions may be asked which may influence the patient's response

Table 4.2 Endodontic procedures and their risks of postoperative bleeding complications.

Risk of postoperative bleeding complications		
Negligible	**Low**	**High**
• Local anaesthetic • Periodontal probing • Placement of rubber dam • Placement of restorations with supragingival margins • Orthograde endodontics	• Incision and drainage of swellings • Restorations with subgingival margins	• Root end surgery

Table 4.3 Current recommendations for management of patients on anticoagulants during high-risk dental procedures.

	Drug	**Current recommendations for dental procedures with a high risk of postoperative bleeding (in consultation with the patient's GP)**
Antiplatelet drugs	• Aspirin • Clopidogrel • Dipyridamole • Prasugrel • Ticagrelor	• Continue without interrupting medication but consider staging extensive procedures and using local haemostats
Vitamin K antagonists	• Warfarin • Acenocoumarol • Phenindione	• Check INR no more than 24 hours before the procedure. • If INR is below 4, continue without interrupting medication but consider staging extensive procedures and using local haemostats • If INR is above 4, delay treatment
Novel oral anticoagulants	• Apixaban • Dabigatran • Rivaroxaban	• Miss morning dose but take usual evening dose • Delay morning dose (if taken in morning). If medication taken in the evening, no action is required

Endodontology at a Glance. First Edition. Alix Davies, Federico Foschi and Shanon Patel. © 2019 John Wiley & Sons, Ltd. Published 2019 by John Wiley & Sons, Ltd.
Companion website: www.wiley.com/go/davies/endodontology

iagnosis of endodontic disease is the process of determining the cause of the patient's signs and symptoms.

In order to reach the correct diagnosis a thorough history must be taken. Extraoral and intraoral examinations are necessary prior to performing additional clinical tests. These are discussed in more detail in Chapters 5–7. The information compiled from the history and examination allows the dentist to develop a differential diagnosis. This is a list of all the possible diagnoses. Special tests then help the clinician to arrive at a definitive diagnosis, although sometimes this is not confirmed until treatment has been completed and the pain resolves, or histology samples have been reported.

Completing a patient history

Presenting symptoms

The patient should be asked why he/she has attended the appointment and be allowed to describe the problem. The clinician can then ask more direct questions to gain additional specific information. A variety of open and closed questions should be used (Table 4.1). The open questions allow the patient to describe the problem without any input bias from the clinician whilst closed questioning allows the consultation to remain focused on the problem, especially when there is limited time. Questioning must establish specific details of the problem and includes the following.

Location of the pain

Can you point to the tooth that is painful?

If the patient cannot localise the exact tooth or area, he/she should be asked to point to the quadrant or side that the pain originates from. When the pain is severe and generalised, the patient should be asked if he/she can remember the site at which the pain was felt at its onset.

Commencement

When did the symptoms first occur?

The pain may coincide with recent dental treatment to a particular tooth. Alternatively, the patient may recollect biting hard onto something. However, care must be taken not to make incorrect conclusions based on this information alone.

Intensity of the pain

On a scale of 1 to 10, with 10 being the most severe, how would you rate your symptoms?

The intensity may change at certain periods such as eating or at night-time and therefore detail should be sought as to any changes in the intensity during a 24-hour period.

Provocation and relief of pain

Does anything worsen or relieve your symptoms?

Patients may describe either biting or temperature changes as being the main initiating factors. Pain on biting or touching a specific tooth suggests acute apical periodontitis or an acute apical abscess. However, the pain may also be caused by a crack.

Prolonged pain in response to hot, cold and sweet suggests inflammation of the pulp.

Relief of the pain may be by non-steroidal anti-inflammatory drugs (NSAIDs), suggesting an inflammatory cause. Cold water may also relieve the pain.

Duration of the pain

How long does the pain linger after it has been provoked?

A pain that lasts for seconds indicates dentine hypersensitivity or a reversible pulpitis. A pain lasting for several minutes after thermal stimuli indicates an irreversible nature.

Relevance of medical history

Medical history questionnaires should be updated at each appointment. Whilst there are no absolute contraindications to provision of root canal treatment, modifications to treatment are sometimes necessary. Some patients have been advised to avoid dental extractions and it may therefore be necessary to attempt to root treat teeth, even when this has a limited prognosis. This may be necessary for patients undergoing intravenous bisphosphonate treatment or head/neck radiotherapy.

Patients with cardiovascular, respiratory and central nervous system disorders may be taking medications that interact with antibiotics, analgesics or anaesthetics used during dental treatment. An up to date list of medications should be taken and checked prior to treatment. Patients with reduced liver or renal function can have reduced ability to metabolise the administered drugs and the dosage may need to be modified.

Pacemakers can interact with older electric pulp testers, electrosurgery equipment and some ultrasonics. A cardiologist's advice would be wise prior to using such equipment. Patients may be taking anticoagulant or antiplatelet drugs. Whilst it is possible to take an international normalised ratio (INR) to assess the risk of bleeding for patients taking warfarin, this is not possible for the novel oral anticoagulants. Therefore, a risk assessment must be taken prior to the procedure (Table 4.2) and, if there is a high risk of bleeding, consultation with the patient's medical practitioner would be advised as the patient's drug schedule may require alteration (Table 4.3).

Known allergies must be assessed; these commonly include various antibiotics and latex. However, anaphylaxis following chlorhexidine use is increasing and dentists must be able to recognise and manage anaphylactic shock.

Patients who are on long-term steroids or who have diabetes have been shown to have a decreased prognosis after root canal treatment, although this is not a contraindication for treatment. Diabetic patients must have their appointment times planned around meals to maintain their correct blood glucose levels.

Pregnant patients may wish to defer non-essential radiographs until after their first trimester for their own piece of mind. However, there is still justification for taking radiographs to assist in pain diagnosis. Endodontic treatment can still be performed but, as always, care must be taken to limit the radiation dose as much as possible. Some patients who are pain free may wish to delay treatment until the second trimester.

5 Examination and special tests

Figure 5.1 (a) Photograph showing sinus tract adjacent to UR4. (b) If gutta percha is placed in the tract, (c) it is easier to identify where the infection originates from.

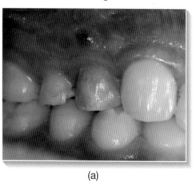

(a)

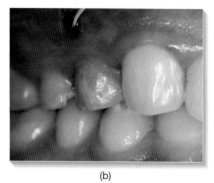

(b)

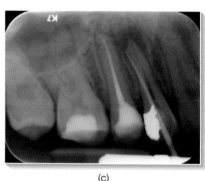

(c)

Figure 5.2 Diagram showing the use of the tooth slooth to identify a cracked cusp.

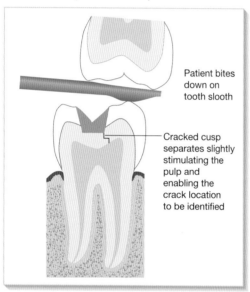

Patient bites down on tooth slooth

Cracked cusp separates slightly stimulating the pulp and enabling the crack location to be identified

Figure 5.3 Diagram showing localised bone loss due to pus discharge and a crack.

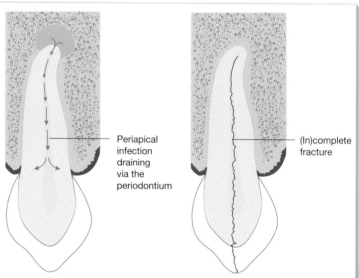

Periapical infection draining via the periodontium

(In)complete fracture

Figure 5.4 A BPE probe should be used to probe the gingival margin to assess for localised pockets.

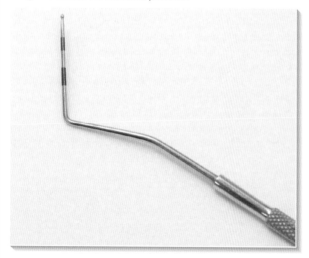

Box 5.1 Characteristics of intraoral swellings.

- Localised or diffuse
- Firm or fluctuant
- Superficial (attached gingiva or alveolar mucosa) or deep (sublingual)
- Is the swelling pointing or draining pus?

Box 5.2 Causes of tooth mobility

- Trauma causing either a subluxation or luxation injury
- Parafunctional habits
- Periodontal disease
- Root fractures
- Rapid orthodontic movement
- Infection of pulpal origin that has tracked into the periodontal ligament space

Endodontology at a Glance. First Edition. Alix Davies, Federico Foschi and Shanon Patel. © 2019 John Wiley & Sons, Ltd. Published 2019 by John Wiley & Sons, Ltd.
Companion website: www.wiley.com/go/davies/endodontology

Extraoral examination

An extraoral examination is necessary to assess for asymmetry caused by swelling and extraoral fistulas. Lymph nodes should also be palpated. Firm tender nodes accompanied by an elevated temperature are indicators of infection. The temporalis and masseter should be assesed for hypertrophy and their origins and attachments should be palpated for tenderness.

The patient's smile line may require assessment as this can influence treatment decisions that involve the gingival margins including replacing anterior crowns or surgical procedures.

Intraoral examination

A complete intraoral soft tissue examination must be performed and any relevant lesions documented and followed up appropriately. Any intraoral swellings should be assessed by visualisation and palpation (Box 5.1). Sinus tracts feature in longstanding infections to provide a drainage pathway for pus. The surface opening (stoma) of the sinus tract can be in the attached gingiva, alveolar mucosa or gingival sulcus. The stoma is commonly, but not always, adjacent to the source of the infection and therefore the origin of the sinus tract should be determined radiographically using gutta percha (Figure 5.1). Palatal fistulae tend to be less visible than buccal ones.

An overall assessment of the restorative state of the teeth is required, noting deficient fillings and caries, prior to assessing the side or quadrant of concern in more detail. The teeth of interest should be assessed visually for tooth wear, large and/or defective fillings, cracks and caries. An estimation of the amount of remaining healthy tooth structure is required. The integrity of any crown margins must also be assessed. Teeth should then undergo various tests to assess tenderness to percussion and palpation, periodontal status and vitality (see Chapter 6). If there is still uncertainty as to the diagnosis, additional tests such as selective anaesthesia may be performed.

When assessing teeth it is important that the contralateral tooth (if asymptomatic and not root filled) is tested first to enable the patient to understand what to expect and what can be considered normal. The occlusion and status of adjacent teeth must also be assessed to determine the strategic importance of maintaining particular teeth. This can affect management decisions of whether to root treat or extract.

Percussion testing

When a patient reports pain on biting, percussion and bite tests are useful aids to localise the problem. Devices such as a tooth slooth (Figure 5.2) allow the clinician to apply pressure to a specific cusp or fossa with more accuracy. Pain on biting occurs either when the pulpal inflammation has extended apically to the periodontal ligament space (acute apical periodontitis) or when there is crack in the tooth. Pain as a result of acute apical periodontitis manifests when pressure is applied, independent of the direction of the percussion. However, a cracked tooth will only be painful when the tooth is percussed in a specific direction. In addition, it is common for pain to be felt when the pressure is released, instead of when it is applied.

Palpation testing

The buccal and, when indicated the lingual/palatal sulci in the area under investigation should be palpated to detect any soft tissue swellings or bony expansion. This should be compared with the contralateral side. The patient should be asked to indicate any areas that feel particularly tender when the pressure is applied. This is an indicator of periradicular inflammation.

Periodontal assessment

Tooth mobility can be assessed by placing the ends of two mirror handles on buccal and lingual aspects of a tooth and applying pressure in various horizontal directions, as well as vertically. Causes of increased mobility are shown in Box 5.2. Periodontal probing around the root surface may identify generalised and localised isolated areas of bone loss. Generalised bone loss is usually of periodontal origin. Localised deep probing depths occur as a result of endodontic infection with pus discharging through the periodontal ligament. A vertical root fracture may also cause a localised narrow periodontal pocket (Figure 5.3). A basic periodontal examination (BPE) probe is best suited to identifying localised periodontal pockets because of its small cross-sectional area (Figure 5.4).

Assessment of cracks

Staining and transillumination can be used to assess cracks. When methylene blue dye is painted on the tooth surface it will penetrate into and stain the cracks. The use of dental loupes or a dental operating microscope will enhance visualisation of the cracks. However, it is difficult to assess the depth of the crack by visualising its surface appearance only, and it may need further investigation.

Test cavities

A test cavity involves preparing a cavity without local anaesthetic to determine if the tooth has an intact pulp. If the bur reaches the dentine without the patient reporting any sensation, the pulp is likely to be necrotic. However, its use is largely historical as the procedure is irreversibly destructive and can be very unpleasant for the patient. It is not a reliable test.

Selective local anaesthesia

Patients with irreversible pulpitis may be unable to identify the offending tooth, or even if the symptoms originate from the maxillary or mandibular arch. Adminstration of local anaesthesia adjacent to the most posterior tooth in the maxillary arch will anaesthetise the upper teeth and, if one of these is the offending tooth, the pain will resolve. If the pain does not subside after a reasonable period of time, the mandibular arch should be anaesthetised. Resolution of the pain would then indicate that the problem is mandibular. This technique is effective in determining whether the problem is localised to the maxillary or mandibular arch but will not determine the specific tooth.

6 Pulp testing

Figure 6.1 Endofrost – this is in the group of refrigerant sprays that are most commonly used.

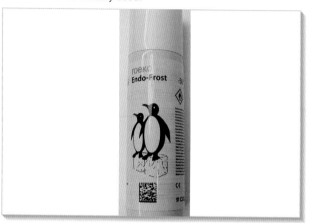

Figure 6.2 Laser Doppler.

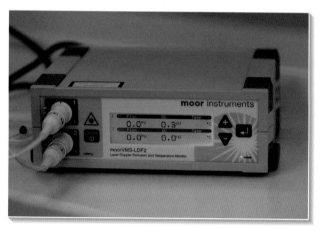

Table 6.1 Advantages and disadvantages of various cold substances used in pulp testing.

Cold pulp tester	Temperature applied to tooth	Advantages	Disadvantages
Cold water	(5–10°C)	• Entire tooth can be cooled down • Can be used to replicate patient symptoms	• Requires single tooth isolation to test • Time consuming
Ethyl chloride	(−4°C)	• Less painful for the patient	• Less rapid cooling and therefore not as sensitive as other cooling methods • Expensive
Refrigerant spray: dichlorodifluoromethane	(−50°C)	• Can produce a response even through restorations and crowns therefore useful when no natural tooth tissue is present • Cheap	• Some of these sprays may contribute to ozone depletion.
tetrafluoroethane	(−26°C)		
Carbon dioxide snow	(−78°C)	• Can produce a response even through restorations and crowns therefore useful when no natural tooth tissue is present • Very rapid pulpal cooling and therefore provides a quick response	• Less readily available • Can be painful for the patient

Box 6.1 Causes of false positive and false negative responses when performing pulp testing.

Causes of false positive responses
• Conduction of the stimulus to adjacent teeth via contacting metallic surfaces (crowns, amalgam restorations)
• Conduction of the stimulus to the gingivae
• Breakdown products of localised pulp necrosis may conduct the stimulus to adjacent pulp tissue
• Multirooted teeth may be partially necrotic but have areas with an intact nerve supply
• Inflamed tissue will still respond to pulp testing – therefore a positive response does not indicate a healthy pulp
• Nervous or young patients are more likely to provide an incorrect response because of the expectation of feeling an unpleasant sensation

Causes of false negative responses
• Recently traumatised teeth may not respond to vitality tests despite having an intact blood supply
• Immature teeth with incomplete root development do not have a mature innervation and may therefore not respond to pulp tests
• Teeth that are undergoing orthodontic movement may not respond reliably to pulp testing
• Patients who are under the influence of narcotics and alcohol may not respond reliably to pulp testing
• Teeth with sclerosed root canals may not respond to pulp testing
• Heavily restored teeth may not respond to pulp testing
• Patients with psychotic disorders may provide irregular results

Endodontology at a Glance. First Edition. Alix Davies, Federico Foschi and Shanon Patel. © 2019 John Wiley & Sons, Ltd. Published 2019 by John Wiley & Sons, Ltd.
Companion website: www.wiley.com/go/davies/endodontology

Pulp tests involving nerve stimulation

The pulp comprises myelinated fibres (mainly Aδ fibres) and unmyelinated C fibres. The Aδ fibres predominantly innervate the dentine tubule endings and the C fibres innervate the body of the pulp. The Aδ fibres are stimulated during pulp testing as they have lower electrical thresholds than the C fibres. Pulp testing usually involves the stimulation of these nerve endings and requires the patient to indicate if they feel the stimulus. The ideal pulp tester would be simple to use, objective, standardised and reproducible. It should not be painful or injurious and should be inexpensive. An ideal test would have high specificity and sensitivity.

When performing a pulp test, a 'control' tooth should be tested first to benchmark a baseline response. This also allows the patient to understand what a 'normal' response is. The ideal tooth is the contralateral tooth providing it is asymptomatic and not root filled. The pulp tester should be placed on the incisal third of anterior teeth and mid third of posterior teeth. Multirooted teeth that give a negative response on one aspect should be tested on the opposite surface to ensure that as much of the pulp as possible has been stimulated. The potentially compromised teeth can then be tested, and the test should be repeated at least twice to confirm the results. It is necessary to isolate teeth to minimise the risk of conduction of the current to adjacent structures. Rubber dam, cotton wool rolls or clear plastic strips can be used.

Thermal pulp testing

Thermal pulp testing relies on the application of heat or cold to a localised part of the tooth. This causes dentinal fluid movement within the dental tubules. The hydrodynamic forces act on the Aδ mechanoreceptors within the dentino-pulp complex. Cold tests include the application of various substances to the tooth surface (Table 6.1; Figure 6.1). The colder the test, the greater the rate of temperature reduction and therefore a greater hydrodynamic force present to stimulate the nerve endings. Cold tests should be applied to the tooth until the patient definitely responds to the stimulus, or for a maximum of 15 seconds. Both buccal and lingual or palatal aspects of the tooth should be assessed.

Heat tests are not as reliable as cold but can be used to try to replicate the patient's pain if the main stimulating factor is hot temperature. Various heat tests include placement of heated gutta percha on to the tooth surface, applying frictional heat from a prophy cup or individually isolating the teeth with rubber dam and submerging them with hot water.

Electric pulp testing

The electric pulp tester comprises a probe that the patient holds, with a tip to touch the tooth that requires testing. When the probe is in contact with the tooth (via a conducting medium such as prophy paste), an electrical circuit is completed and current will flow. A pulsating electrical stimulus is produced. This is initially of low intensity which gradually increases. It produces an ionic shift in the dentinal tubule fluid which will depolarise the Aδ nerve endings.

Thermal and electrical pulp testing are subjective tests and provide information about the nerve supply only, not the more important vascular supply. These tests are neither particularly sensitive nor specific, with false positive and false negative results commonly being produced (Box 6.1). Whilst pulp testing is a valuable test, no single technique can reliably interpret and diagnose all pulpal conditions and the results should always be considered along with the history, examination, other special tests and radiographs.

Alternative pulp tests that assess the blood supply

Crown surface temperature

This test requires isolation and cooling of the tooth in question along with a suitable control (i.e. healthy contralateral tooth). Thermographic imaging then determines the rate at which the teeth warm up. Teeth with an intact vascular supply warm faster than non-vital teeth. This method is advantageous in that it measures the blood supply rather than the nerve supply. However, the patient is required to rest for a period of time before the test is performed, causing it to be very time consuming and impractical.

Laser Doppler (Figure 6.2)

Light is emitted that scatters when it hits moving objects such as red blood cells. This shift in frequency of the scattered light is measured to determine the blood flow through the pulp. If there is no blood flow, there will be no shift in frequency. This technique is more reliable than pulp sensitivity testing in assessing and following up the pulp status of traumatised teeth. However, the device is technique sensitive and requires rubber dam and a putty matrix to ensure the probe is placed in the identical position at each follow-up visit. The equipment is also relatively expensive.

Pulse oximetry

This test measures oxygen saturation levels in the pulpal blood supply. However, although it has the potential to assess blood flow in traumatised teeth, it has not been successfully adapted for dental use.

7 Radiographic imaging for endodontics

Figure 7.1 Diagram of paralleling technique showing how the film is placed parallel to the tooth, and the X-ray tube head perpendicular to both.

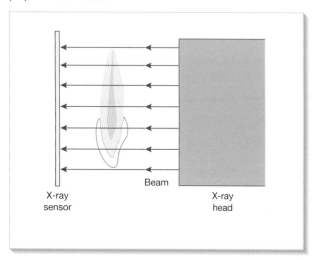

Beam

X-ray sensor

X-ray head

Figure 7.2 Diagram of bisected angle technique. The angle between the plane of the tooth and film is bisected, and the X-ray tube head is aimed perpendicular to this.

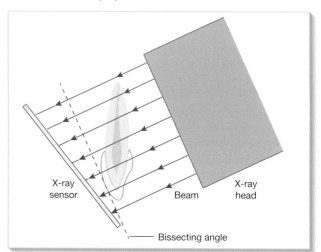

X-ray sensor

Beam

X-ray head

Bissecting angle

Figure 7.3 (a) Periapical radiograph of UR6 showing a fractured file in the mesio-buccal root. The presence of a periapical area is not obvious. (b) Reconstructed CBCT image clearly shows the extent of the periapical area.

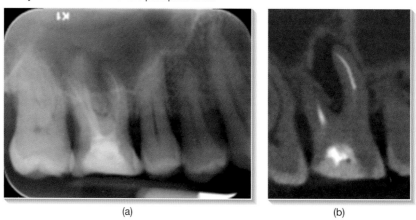

(a)

(b)

Figure 7.4 (a) Periapical radiograph of the LL2 showing a small resorptive defect. (b) Reconstructed sagittal and axial CBCT screenshots of LL1 showing the labio-lingual extent of the resorption. Source: A. Davies. The benefits and limitations of CBCT. *Endodontic Practice* 2016:19;3. Reproduced with permission.

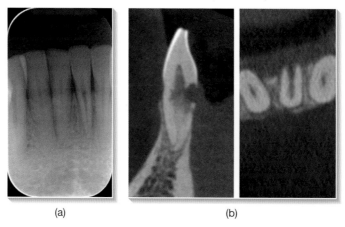

(a)

(b)

Endodontology at a Glance. First Edition. Alix Davies, Federico Foschi and Shanon Patel. © 2019 John Wiley & Sons, Ltd. Published 2019 by John Wiley & Sons, Ltd.
Companion website: www.wiley.com/go/davies/endodontology

Periapical radiography in diagnosis and management of endodontic disease

A periapical radiograph aims to show the entire tooth and surrounding periapical tissues. The film should be used with a beam aiming device. It should be positioned as close to the tooth as possible, and ideally parallel with it. The parallelling technique is the most reproducible (Figure 7.1), but if it is not possible to place the film in this position a bisecting angle technique should be adopted (Figure 7.2).

Root canal infection causes inflammation at the root apex resulting in the production of inflammatory mediators, some of which cause osteoclast recruitment and bone resorption. This resorption produces a bony defect which absorbs less radiation and consequently shows as a dark area on the radiographic film. Acute inflammation can result in accumulation of exudate in the periodontal ligament, causing it to appear slightly widened on a periapical radiograph. However, many cases show no evident change. As inflammation persists, the lamina dura and then cancellous bone are lost. This area can be surrounded by dense sclerotic bone known as sclerosing osteitis.

If there is a sinus tract present, its origin can be determined using the gutta percha tracer technique. A gutta percha cone should be placed in the sinus tract and advanced until resistance is felt. A periapical radiograph should be taken with this in place to show the gutta percha point tracking to the source of the infection (see Chapter 5).

Periapical radiography is considered the gold standard view for assessing teeth with endodontic disease as it provides an overview of the marginal bone levels, restorative status of the tooth and root canal morphology. It can also demonstrate the presence of periapical radiolucencies. It is inexpensive, widely available and can be understood by both dental professionals and patients. The images produced are of good resolution.

Limitations of periapical radiography in the diagnosis of endodontic disease

A single radiograph is limited in its diagnostic ability because of anatomical noise from adjacent structures including the maxillary sinus, zygomatic arch and inferior dental nerve. In multirooted teeth, the buccal and lingual or palatal roots may be superimposed, preventing visualisation and appreciation of the entire root canal anatomy. Severe canal curvature with buccolingual orientation may be underestimated. Visualisation is even harder if root filling is present as the radiopacity of this can mask any untreated canals. Parallel periapical radiographs are bidimensional, only providing information about the tooth and periapical tissues in the mesiodistal plane. Appreciation of the true size of periapical radiolucencies is therefore unknown.

A periapical radiolucency is often only identified after bone loss has extended to the thick cortical plates and therefore many teeth with periapical bone loss confined to the cancellous bone may be missed.

Cone beam computed tomography in endodontic diagnosis and management

Cone beam computed tomography (CBCT) produces three-dimensional scans of the maxillofacial region with a single orbit of the cone-shaped beam and radiographic detector. The three-dimensional scan allows assessment of the anatomy of the tooth, surrounding dentoalveolar anatomy and any pathology to be assessed in multiple planes with the removal of anatomical noise. CBCT now has a major role in the diagnosis and management of endodontic problems and is to be recommended in the following cases:

- Diagnosis of radiographic signs of periapical pathosis when signs or symptoms are non-specific.
- Assessment and management of complex dentoalveolar trauma.
- Assessment of complex root canal anatomy in teeth requiring non surgical endodontic treatment.
- Assessment of complex root canal anatomy in teeth planned for non-surgical retreatment.
- Assessment of endodontic treatment complications such as fractured files or perforations when existing radiographic views have provided insufficient information.
- Assessment of root resorption that appears to be potentially treatable.
- Presurgical assessment prior to complex periradicular surgery.

CBCT images are of a lower resolution than conventional radiographs. High-density structures such as crowns, restorations or metal posts affect the image, as a result of scattering, producing images of minimal diagnostic value. CBCT is relatively expensive.

Risks of ionising radiation

Both periapical radiographs and CBCT use ionising radiation. It is essential that patients are exposed to the lowest reasonably achievable dose. The effective dose of a periapical radiograph is approximately 5 μSv, depending on the area of interest and the type of collimation used. The effective dose of a small field of view CBCT ranges from 13–100 μSv, depending on the scanner, area of interest and the size of the field of view. CBCT should therefore only be used in situations where information from conventional radiography does not yield adequate information to allow appropriate management of the patient. For endodontic purposes, the smallest possible field of view (FOV) should be used.

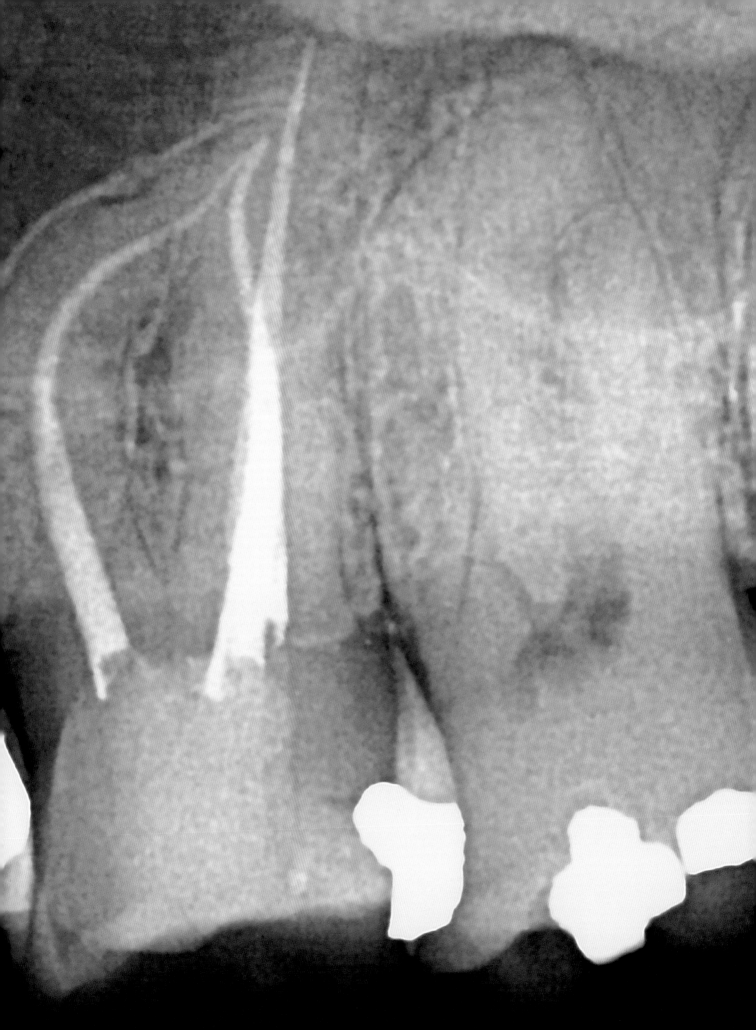

Endodontic therapy

Part 3

Chapters

8 Vital pulp therapy

Figure 8.1 Histological zones within the pulp.

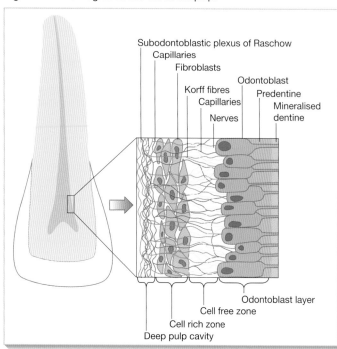

- Subodontoblastic plexus of Raschow
- Capillaries
- Fibroblasts
- Korff fibres
- Capillaries
- Nerves
- Odontoblast
- Predentine
- Mineralised dentine
- Odontoblast layer
- Cell free zone
- Cell rich zone
- Deep pulp cavity

Figure 8.2 Positions of secondary dentine, tertiary dentine and sclerotic dentine.

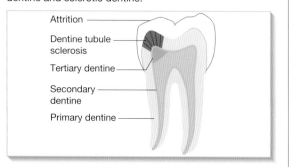

- Attrition
- Dentine tubule sclerosis
- Tertiary dentine
- Secondary dentine
- Primary dentine

Figure 8.3 Histopathological zones of dentine caries.

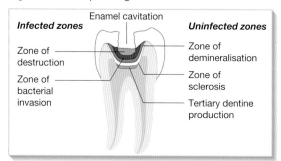

Enamel cavitation

Infected zones
- Zone of destruction
- Zone of bacterial invasion

Uninfected zones
- Zone of demineralisation
- Zone of sclerosis
- Tertiary dentine production

Figure 8.4 Stages of vital pulp therapy, (the use of rubber dam is essential).

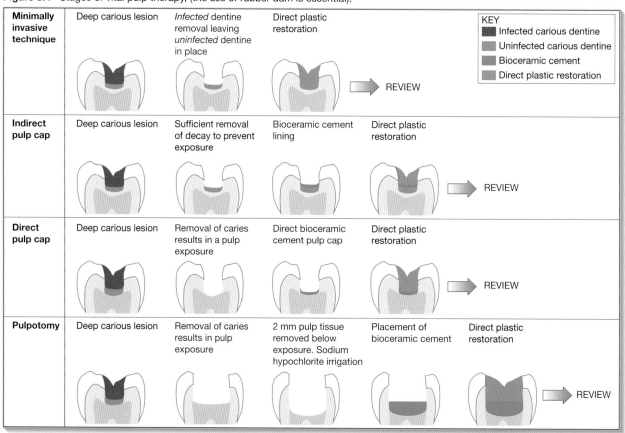

Minimally invasive technique	Deep carious lesion	*Infected* dentine removal leaving *uninfected* dentine in place	Direct plastic restoration		REVIEW
Indirect pulp cap	Deep carious lesion	Sufficient removal of decay to prevent exposure	Bioceramic cement lining	Direct plastic restoration	REVIEW
Direct pulp cap	Deep carious lesion	Removal of caries results in a pulp exposure	Direct bioceramic cement pulp cap	Direct plastic restoration	REVIEW
Pulpotomy	Deep carious lesion	Removal of caries results in pulp exposure	2 mm pulp tissue removed below exposure. Sodium hypochlorite irrigation	Placement of bioceramic cement	Direct plastic restoration	REVIEW

KEY
- Infected carious dentine
- Uninfected carious dentine
- Bioceramic cement
- Direct plastic restoration

Endodontology at a Glance. First Edition. Alix Davies, Federico Foschi and Shanon Patel. © 2019 John Wiley & Sons, Ltd. Published 2019 by John Wiley & Sons, Ltd.
Companion website: www.wiley.com/go/davies/endodontology

Role of the dental pulp after tooth development is complete

The pulp chamber and root canals contain the dental pulp. This contains four histologically distinguishable zones (Figure 8.1). The odontoblast outer layer of the pulp is responsible for dentine formation; a healthy pulp is essential for tooth development. Once root development is complete, the pulp's function is mainly a protective one.

Secondary dentine is produced by odontoblasts during the lifespan of the tooth. This makes the tooth more resilient. Tertiary dentine can additionally be laid down at specific sites in response to potential damage caused by stimuli such as caries or attrition (Figure 8.2). These potentially damaging stimuli also cause dentine sclerosis. Hydroxyapatite crystals are secreted by the odontoblasts and precipitate in the dentine tubules, reducing their permeability and delaying the ingress of bacteria and their toxins.

The dental pulp is richly innervated. Nerve fibres enter the pulp through the apical foramen to form a subodontoblastic plexus. A few axons pass between the odontoblasts to enter the dentine tubules. These can depolarise in response to fluid changes in the tubule and provide a warning of noxious stimuli that can be associated with tissue damage.

The dentinal tubules contain fluid produced by ultrafiltration from the pulpal capillaries. This can dilute any toxins to reduce their damaging effects. The hydrostatic pressure is highest at the pulpal aspect of the tubule and the outwards force therefore minimises the invasion of microorganisms for a finite period. The blood supply to the pulp is necessary to transport immune cells and inflammatory mediators to the area and to dilute and remove damaging agents, therefore resisting infection for as long as possible.

Benefits of maintaining a vital pulp

Root treated teeth have a lower survival rate than their untreated counterparts. This may be due to inadequate disinfection resulting in a persistent infection, or reinfection of the root canal system from coronal microleakage. In addition, root treated teeth are weaker and consequently are at increased risk of fracture (see Chapter 26). Root canal treatment is costly and time consuming to perform, as is the placement of a cuspal coverage restoration.

Performing root canal treatment on an immature tooth has the added challenge of poor patient compliance. Immature root apices make compaction of the root filling more difficult. Incomplete dentine formation results in thinner roots, increasing the risk of tooth fracture. If the vitality of a tooth can be maintained, secondary dentine deposition will continue, thereby reinforcing the root and reducing its risk of fracture.

Vital pulp therapy

A cavitated carious lesion progressing through dentine shows various histological zones from demineralisation to destruction (Figure 8.3). As it nears the pulp, reversible and, eventually, irreversible pulpal inflammation develops. However, as microorganisms are not at the deepest part of a carious lesion, superficial infected caries can be removed, leaving the semi-mineralised non-infected carious dentine behind. If the lesion is sealed to prevent further bacterial ingress, it may be possible to preserve vitality of the pulp rather than resort to root canal treatment. This is the basis of pulp capping (Figure 8.4). This procedure can only be performed in teeth that are responsive to pulp vitality testing and are asymptomatic, or have symptoms suggestive of reversible pulpitis. Pulp capping and pulpotomies are also indicated in traumatic dental injuries (see Chapter 32).

Stepwise excavation is not discussed in this chapter, as the authors believe it is now an outdated treatment concept.

- **Indirect pulp capping** involves removal of as much of the carious lesion as possible but leaving an intact thin layer of dentine over the roof of the pulp chamber.
- **Direct pulp capping** includes the placement of a bioceramic cement, e.g. Mineral Trioxide Aggregate (MTA), Biodentine directly on a pulpal exposure. The cavity is then restored with a direct plastic restoration.
- **Pulpotomy** involves removal of at least 2mm of exposed pulp tissue with a sterile diamond bur in a fast headpiece with copious water spray. The exposed pulp wound is then restored with a bioceramic cement and subsequently restored with a direct plastic restoration.

Pulp preservation is recommended wherever possible, especially in teeth with immature roots. Treatment should always be carried out under rubber dam, and the cavity disinfected with sodium hypochlorite prior to placement of the bioceramic cement.

9 Root canal morphology

Figure 9.1 Outline forms for access cavities for each tooth.

Maxillary teeth	1	2	3	4	5	6	7
Root length (mm)	23	22	26	21	21	22	20
Number of canals	1	1	1	1–5% 2–90% (B, P) 3–5% (MB, DB, P)	1–75% 2–25% (B, P)	3–40% (MB, DB, P) 4–60% (MB1, MB2, DB, P)	3–60% (MB, DB, P) 4–40% (MB1, MB2, DB, P)
Features	• Access starts at cingulum and extends towards the incisal edge • Incisors have 2 pulp horns so access must be triangular • The canine only has one pulp horn so access can be rounder • Apex of lateral incisor curves palatally			• Access should be intiated at the mid point of the central groove and then widened bucco-palatally • If only one canal is present it will be in the midline – if it is not, then another canal will be present • Canals often converge at the apex		• Outline access cavity is rhomboidal • Palatal root canal often the largest and easiest to locate • MB2 located between MB1 and palatal root canal • Increased likelihood of fusion of root canals in 2nd and 3rd molars to 1 buccal and 1palatal	

Buccal

Palatal

Lingual

Buccal

Mandibular teeth	1	2	3	4	5	6	7
Root length (mm)	21	21	24	22	22	21	20
Number of canals	1–60% 2–40% (B, L)	1–60% 2–40% (B, L)	1–90% 2–10% (B, L)	1–75% 2–25% (B, L)	1–90% 2–10% (B, L)	3–65% (MB, ML, D) 4–35% (ML, MB, DL, DB)	3–90% (MB, ML, D) 2–10% (M, D)
Features	• Access starts at the base of the cingulum • In incisors this needs to extend close to the incisal edge to confirm the presence or absence of a lingual canal			• Access starts in midpoint of central groove		• Mesial root canal orifices are found below respective cusp tips • If one distal canal is present, it is in the centre. If it is not centred, another canal should be searched for • 2nd and 3rd molars may show fusion of canals into 1 mesial and 1 distal canal	

B - buccal, P - palatal, MB - mesiobuccal, DB - distobuccal, MB1 - first mesiobuccal, MB2 - second mesiobuccal, L - lingual, ML - mesiolingual, D - distal, DL - distolingual

Endodontology at a Glance. First Edition. Alix Davies, Federico Foschi and Shanon Patel. © 2019 John Wiley & Sons, Ltd. Published 2019 by John Wiley & Sons, Ltd.
Companion website: www.wiley.com/go/davies/endodontology

Successful root canal treatment requires thorough disinfection and obturation of the entire root canal system. This can be challenging as the root canal system comprises a range of canal configurations based on the tooth type and also on individual variability. Prior to starting any root canal treatment, it is important to be familiar with the normal root canal anatomy for each tooth (Figure 9.1). Full assessment of the periapical radiograph is necessary to gain information about the anatomy of the specific tooth undergoing treatment. If further information is required, supplemental parallax radiographs or CBCT reconstructed images are often beneficial. A well-designed access cavity (see Chapter 10) and the use of magnification are essential to determine canal entrances and other anatomical features such as bifurcation of canals.

Maxillary incisors

Centrals are on average 23 mm long and the laterals are 21–22 mm. The lateral incisor may have variations to include an extra root, dens invaginatus, gemination or fusion. Trauma can cause early devitalisation of these teeth, preventing full root development and therefore producing infected necrotic teeth with blunderbuss apices and thin dentine walls (see Chapter 27).

Dens invaginatus is a dental malformation, probably resulting from an infolding of the dental papilla during tooth development before mineralisation. Incidence is reported as between 0.25 and 10%. Lateral incisors are most commonly affected and occur bilaterally in 43% of cases. There are various forms of dens invaginatus. The enamel lining of the invagination is often incomplete and can contain channels that communicate with the pulp. This can facilitate the entry of microorganisms to the pulp. Pulpal necrosis often occurs within a few years of eruption and prior to the completion of root development. CBCT is often necessary to assess the invagination to ascertain appropriate management.

Maxillary canine

This is the longest tooth (average 26 mm) and usually occurs with a single canal.

Maxillary premolars

These teeth have various root canal configurations. Occasionally, a premolar has three root canals in two or three roots. This is indicated if there is a disparity in the buccal and palatal root lengths, or a buccal indentation can be probed. Premolars show a high incidence of lateral canals near the apical foramen. Their average lengths are 21 mm for first maxillary premolars and 21.5 mm for second maxillary premolars.

Maxillary molars

First maxillary molars usually have three roots and three or four root canals. An additional mesiobuccal (MB2) canal is reported to be present in up to 90% of cases. It either joins the first mesiobuccal (MB1) or occurs as a separate canal. The distal and palatal canals are almost always single canals, the palatal root is the longest. Second maxillary molars are slightly smaller and the three roots are more likely to be fused. There is an additional MB2 canal in 40% of teeth. Maxillary third molars are very variable and have separate or fused roots of any configuration.

Mandibular central and lateral incisors

These teeth are on average 21 mm although the central incisor is often shorter than the lateral incisor. The presence of two canals (labial and lingual) occurs in up to 40% of teeth. However, in most cases these converge into one canal at the apex. Only about 5% of incisors have two canals with separate apical foramina.

Mandibular canine

This has an average length of 22.5 mm and an incidence of 14% with two separate canals, although only about 5% have separate apical foramina.

Mandibular premolar

First and second premolars are usually single rooted with only a very low proportion (< 10%) having a second canal. The presence of multiple canals has been reported. These can be very difficult to treat as they can bifurcate in the apical third and so are difficult to access.

Mandibular molars

These teeth usually have one mesial and one distal root. The molar is of average length (21 mm) and has two mesial canals and one distal canal. A second distal canal can be identified in about 35% of cases and these often converge at the apex. The two mesial canals unite in one apical foramen in about 40% of cases. An additional third canal is identified in the mesial root in 1–7% of cases.

Second molars are slightly smaller in length (21 mm). They show a higher incidence of mesial canal convergence; 90% will have one distal canal. Third molars can be similar to second molars but are very variable and have separate or fused roots of any configuration.

Mandibular molars can have an additional distolingual root (radix entomolaris). Its occurrence is less than 5% in Caucasians but it occurs in 30% of the Chinese population. The orifice will be positioned mesiolingually from the main canal.

Another anatomical variant found in second canals (especially in patients of Asiatic origin) are molars with C-shaped canals. These require a good access cavity, lots of irrigation with ultrasonic files and obturation using a warm vertical condensation technique.

10 Access cavity design

Figure 10.1 A tooth once all fillings have been removed revealing a large crack (arrow). This tooth is unrestorable. Source: S. Patel & J. Rhodes. A practical guide to endodontic access cavity preparation in molar teeth. *British Dental Journal* 2007:203;133–140. Reproduced with permission.

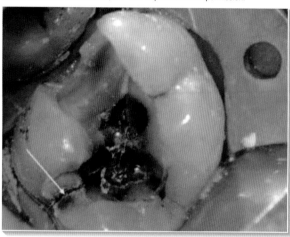

Figure 10.2 Essential burs required for endodontic procedures. (a) Transmetal bur. (b) Coarse long diamond bur. (c) Rosehead bur. (d) Endo Z bur.

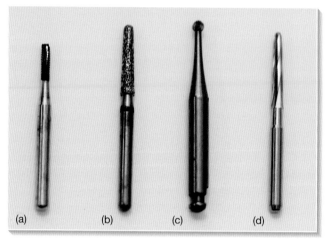

(a)   (b)   (c)   (d)

Figure 10.3 (a) Lower molars usually have one distal oval canal which is in the midline. However there may be two separate canals. If the canal is smaller, round and not in the midline, further exploration is required to locate a second distal canal on the contralateral side of the tooth (b).

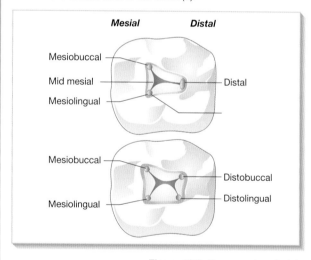

Figure 10.4 (a) File in canal showing the overhang interfering with straight line access. (b) The overhang has been removed to facilitate the required access. (c) Heat-treated NiTi file systems may be precurved allowing them to access areas where straight line access may be difficult to achieve.

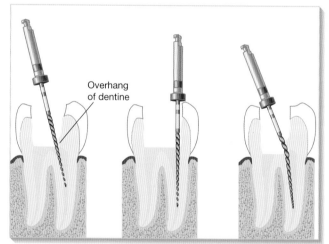

Figure 10.5 Errors such as ledging, zipping and perforations.

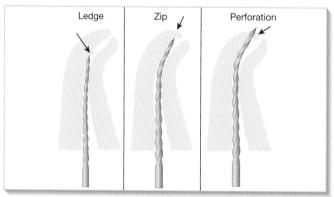

Endodontology at a Glance. First Edition. Alix Davies, Federico Foschi and Shanon Patel. © 2019 John Wiley & Sons, Ltd. Published 2019 by John Wiley & Sons, Ltd.
Companion website: www.wiley.com/go/davies/endodontology

Aim of the access cavity

Good access to the root canal system is important to facilitate identification of the root canal orifices. It should also maximise straight line access into the canals. This allows for more effective root canal debridement and reduces the risk of complications. An effective access cavity will also reduce the risk of leaving undercuts in the pulp chamber that may harbour pulp remnants and residual bacteria.

Stages in access cavity preparation

Removal of restorations and caries

The outline of the access cavity is often dictated by the presence of restorations and/or decay. All restorations, including crowns, should be removed whenever possible. Many older fillings have secondary caries or microleakage, even if they cannot be identified preoperatively. Removal of all the restorations enables a more thorough assessment of restorability which affects management decisions regarding retention of the tooth and, if it is salvageable, deciding on the method by which it will be restored. Identification of cracks is also easier if all the fillings are removed (Figure 10.1). Restoration removal improves visibility and orientation, therefore minimising the risk of procedural errors such as perforations. Apex locators and working length determination are more accurate in the absence of metallic restorations.

Restoration removal can be performed with diamond burs. Rosehead, round tungsten carbide or stainless steel burs are required to remove any caries. Crown removal requires coarse diamond burs to cut through the porcelain. Sectioning of the metal is more efficient with a tungsten carbide bur such as the transmetal bur (Figure 10.2).

The tooth should then be restored with a pre-endodontic restoration to allow rubber dam placement and to create a reservoir to allow retention of irrigating solutions. Glass ionomer or composite are suitable materials for this interim restoration.

Preparation of the outline form

Once the restorations and caries have been removed, an outline should be cut to remove any remaining enamel and dentine over the pulp chamber. There must be adequate extension of the canal outline where necessary to facilitate location of additional lingual canals in lower incisors and distolingual canals in a lower molar.

Penetration of the pulp chamber

The pulp chamber should be penetrated at its largest point. This is centrally for anterior teeth and lower premolars, aiming towards the palatal root for upper premolars and molars and towards the distal root for lower molars. A high speed handpiece is most effective for this and the operator should feel the sudden decrease in resistance to cutting as they 'drop into the pulp'. If the pulp is not located, the operator should re-evaluate the angle of the bur and, if necessary, take angled 'check' radiographs to assess the position relative to the pulp chamber. Magnification is essential, (e.g. loupes or a dental operating microscope). Care must be taken to not cut too deeply and risk perforating the floor. Measurements of the distance of the pulp chamber roof from the cusp tips can be taken, and the bur should cut no deeper than this. Secondary and tertiary dentine deposition can significantly alter the volume of the pulp chamber; accurate observation of the preoperative X-ray can reveal this.

Removal of the pulp chamber roof and canal identification

A safe non-end cutting bur such as the Endo Z bur (Figure 10.2) should be used to remove the remaining pulp chamber roof and modify the axial walls. If the pulp chamber has receded or is calcified, access burs such as the goose neck bur may be useful. Ultrasonic tips are also often effective in these cases. Once accessed, the pulp chamber should be irrigated with hypochlorite. Calcifications in the pulp chamber should also be removed with ultrasonics to maximise visualisation. The canal entrances can then be located, positioned at the junction of the angles of the walls and floor of the pulp chamber. In upper premolars and lower molars, the canals are symmetrical. If this is not the case, further exploration is needed to identify an additional canal (Figure 10.3). The MB2 canal of an upper molar is usually positioned medially and close to the mesiobuccal canal, on a line that intersects the mesiobuccal and palatal canals.

Straight line access

Overhangs and ledges should be removed from the axial walls and an explorer should be placed in each canal to confirm that straight line access has been achieved (Figure 10.4). This is necessary to prevent errors such as ledging, zipping and perforations (Figure 10.5). Straight line access reduces the torque placed on the files, lowering their risk of fracture.

Placing of rubber dam

The timing of rubber dam placement depends on the ease of access cavity preparation and confidence and preference of the operator. Some clinicians prefer to place it at the beginning whilst others prefer to delay until the access cavity has been prepared. The latter can help with orientation of the tooth and minimises the risk of perforation as well as enabling 'check' radiographs to be taken without risk of superimposition of the rubber dam clamps. However, preparation without rubber dam can also allow microbial contamination of the root canal system and therefore it should be placed as soon as possible. Irrigation with sodium hypochlorite should not be performed until the rubber dam is in place.

11 Mechanical preparation of the root canals

Figure 11.1 The file sequence for manual preparation (left to right), coronal, apical and stepback preparation).

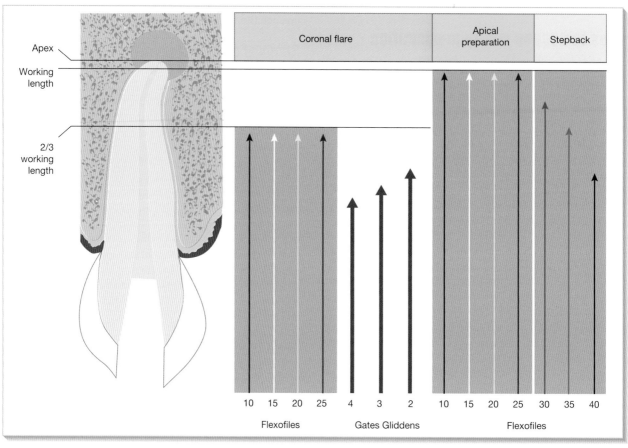

Figure 11.2 The optimal positioning of a Gates Glidden drill to reduce the risk of furcal perforation.

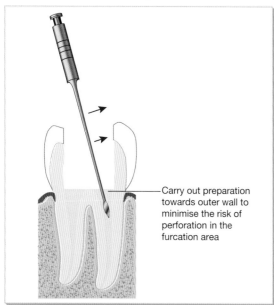

Carry out preparation towards outer wall to minimise the risk of perforation in the furcation area

Figure 11.3 Apical anatomy of the tooth. The canal should be prepared and filled to the apical constriction (working length) which is usually 0.5–1 mm short of the apical foramen).

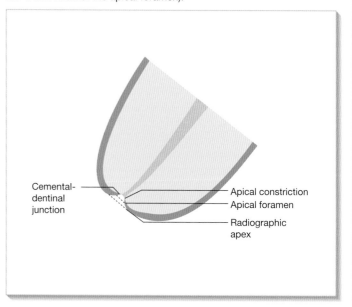

Cemental-dentinal junction

Apical constriction
Apical foramen
Radiographic apex

Endodontology at a Glance. First Edition. Alix Davies, Federico Foschi and Shanon Patel. © 2019 John Wiley & Sons, Ltd. Published 2019 by John Wiley & Sons, Ltd.
Companion website: www.wiley.com/go/davies/endodontology

Root canal instrumentation aims to:
- Remove the bulk of debris from the canals.
- Create adequate space for irrigants and medicaments to penetrate the root canal system.
- Create a suitable resistant form for root canal obturation.

Instrumentation can be performed by hand, by mechanised instruments (rotary or reciprocating) or a combination of the two. Various techniques have been advocated for manual preparation of the root canals. The most commonly adopted manual technique involves a crown down approach, followed by the apical preparation with the step back technique.

Crown down technique

It is recommended that the coronal two-thirds of the canal are opened prior to instrumentation of the apical portion. This can be accomplished by hand files and Gates Glidden drills or rotary instruments (Figure 11.1).

Coronal flaring is advantageous as it provides straighter access to the apical region, thus minimising the force placed on the files and so reducing the risk of complications such as ledges, zipping and perforations. It also lowers the stress placed on instruments, thereby lessening their risk of fracture. Infected teeth contain the bulk of microorganisms in the coronal portion. Enlargement of the coronal canal allows a reservoir of irrigant to be introduced. Irrigants not only help cleanse the canals, but also reduce the risk of blockage formation from compaction of dry dentinal debris. Bacterial extrusion is also reduced when flaring the coronal third of the canal first.

However, the coronal flare can be associated with increased dentine removal which, if excessive, can weaken the tooth and predispose it to fracture. Incorrect positioning of Gates Glidden drills can result in perforation errors. This is avoided by directing the Gates Glidden burs away from the furcation area (Figure 11.2).

Apical preparation

Once the coronal two-thirds have been instrumented, a fine file (size 8) should pass to the apex of the canal. The position of the apical foramen can be confirmed with an apex locator (see Chapter 15) and from this, the working length should be determined (Figure 11.3). Files of increasing apical sizes should be then introduced to the working length until a file of minimum size 25 can reach the working length. Larger canals such as central incisors, distal roots of lower molars and palatal roots of upper molars can require instrumentation to a file gauge of a significantly larger size.

Patency filling

During root canal preparation, dentine chips produced by instrumentation and fragments of apical pulp tissue can become compacted into the apical area. This may cause a blockage of the canal and interfere with the working length. Patency filing involves the passage of a small file (#8) through the apical constriction during apical instrumentation and aims to reduce the risk of blockage. Removal of this debris rather than creating a dentine plug and forcing a file through the apex helps decrease the level of post-endodontic pain. Irrigants may not reach the apical third as they form a vapour lock (air bubble) at the end of the canal. Patency filing may increase penetration of irrigants to this area by breaking up the existing bubble of air, thereby maximising disinfection.

Step back technique

This technique was originally designed to create a tapered preparation using a nearly parallel instrument whilst avoiding preparation errors in curved canals. It involves the placement of files of increasing apical gauges at successively decreasing working lengths. This produces an apical preparation with an increased taper enabling increased penetration of irrigating solutions.

Rotary instrumentation

Nickel titanium rotary instruments were introduced in the 1990s and have since become very popular in root canal preparation (see Chapter 14). A major advantage of the nickel–titanium alloy is its superelasticity and its ability to retain flexibility despite the increased taper. This has resulted in the development of groups of instruments that have a taper of two to six times that of an ISO standardized 2% taper file. Certain files are also characterised by an increasing or variable taper. Rotary instruments allow the canal to be prepared more quickly, with less operator fatigue. The increased apical taper enhances irrigation of the apical portion. Canals prepared with rotary instruments have shown improved shaping, and in some cases fewer procedural errors and less debris extrusion. However, rotary instrumentation has not shown significantly improved outcomes compared with hand instrumentation.

Potential problems with nickel titanium instruments include their liability to undergo breakage. Rotary files are significantly more expensive than stainless steel hand files. Concerns have also been raised about the production of microcracks at the apex of teeth prepared with rotary instruments, although the evidence for this and its clinical significance is conflicting.

12 Irrigation

Figure 12.1 Syringe components and delivery, note the side venting needle.

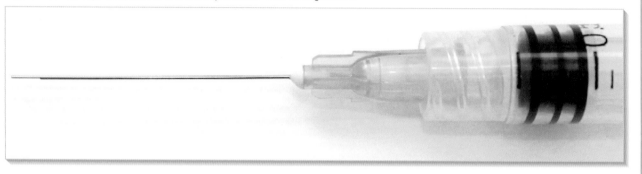

Figure 12.2 Manually activated irrigation.

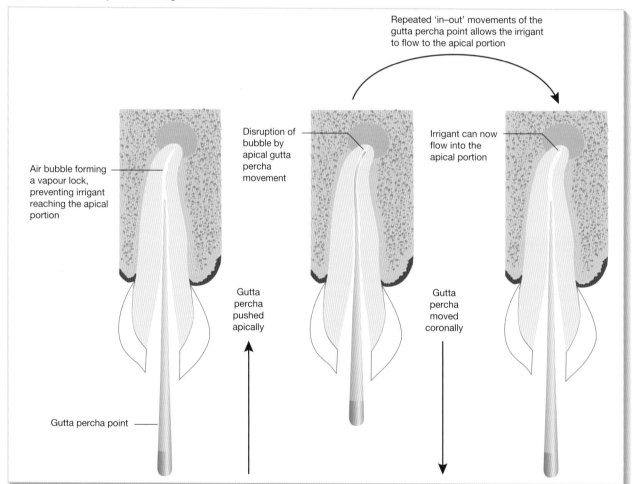

Repeated 'in–out' movements of the gutta percha point allows the irrigant to flow to the apical portion

Air bubble forming a vapour lock, preventing irrigant reaching the apical portion

Disruption of bubble by apical gutta percha movement

Irrigant can now flow into the apical portion

Gutta percha pushed apically

Gutta percha moved coronally

Gutta percha point

Box 12.1 Properties of an ideal root canal irrigating solution.

- Bactericidal with broad spectrum antimicrobial activity
- Ability to dissolve organic necrotic debris
- Ability to remove the inorganic component of the smear layer
- Ability to lubricate the canals
- Non-irritating to the healthy periapical tissues

Endodontology at a Glance. First Edition. Alix Davies, Federico Foschi and Shanon Patel. © 2019 John Wiley & Sons, Ltd. Published 2019 by John Wiley & Sons, Ltd.
Companion website: www.wiley.com/go/davies/endodontology

The primary aim of root canal treatment is to reduce the bacterial load in the root canals to allow the body response to prevent, or in cases of established cases, eliminate endodontic disease. Mechanical instrumentation alone is inadequate for disinfecting the root canals and therefore root canal irrigants must also be used. The properties of an ideal irrigant are shown in Box 12.1.

Irrigants for disinfecting the root canal

Currently used irrigants include mixtures of sodium hypochlorite (NaOCl), ethylenediamine tetra-acetic acid (EDTA), chlorhexidine and iodine potassium iodide. Hydrogen peroxide use is not advised because of concerns over surgical emphysema.

NaOCl is considered the most suitable endodontic irrigant. It can dissolve organic material and possesses broad spectrum antimicrobial activity. However, it only weakly removes the inorganic component of the smear layer.

NaOCl has been used in concentrations from 0.5% to 6%. Low concentrations dissolve the necrotic pulp tissue and destroy the bacteria that they are in direct contact with. Higher concentrations have a more rapid effect; however, they can also irritate the healthy periapical tissue. This can result in more periapical tissue damage if the solution is extruded through the apex. Temperature can also increase the effectiveness of NaOCl in dissolving the organic material.

Complications associated with the use of NaOCl include damage to clothing (bleach spots), splashes into the eyes of the operator or patient, injection through the apical foramen into the periapical tissues or into the maxillary sinus (see Chapter 21).

EDTA may be used alongside NaOCl. It only has limited antimicrobial activity but is effective in dissolving the inorganic component of the smear layer, therefore exposing the dentine tubules. This complements the action of NaOCl, enabling it to act on bacteria on the root dentine surface or within the tubule orifices. A final irrigation with 17% EDTA for 1 minute followed by a rinse with NaOCL is commonly recommended to remove the smear layer prior to obturating the canals. Longer exposures can cause excessive removal of peritubular and intertubular dentine.

Chlorhexidine has broad spectrum antibacterial action. It is dicationic and can therefore attach to the negatively charged bacterial cell membranes to cause cell lysis. It can simultaneously bind to the hydroxyapatite to increase its substantivity. Chlorhexidine has therefore been advocated by some as a final rinse agent in its 2% concentration. However, it should not be used simultaneously with NaOCl as the two chemicals react together to produce an insoluble complex that can interfere with further instrumentation and irrigation. Chlorhexidine cannot dissolve organic tissue and therefore is not recommended for use in isolation of other irrigants. There are also increasing reports of allergy to chlorhexidine.

Methods of irrigation for disinfection of the root canal

Syringe delivery involves the use of a Luer lock syringe with a side venting needle (Figure 12.1). It facilitates the flushing of larger particles of debris and enables the irrigant to have direct contact with microorganisms in the areas reached by the needle tip. However, fluid exchange only takes place 1–1.5 mm beyond the needle tip. Whilst larger gauge needles allow the irrigant to be flushed and replenished more quickly, their diameter minimises the depth to which they can enter the root canal. A finer gauge needle improves the exchange of irrigant in the apical portion of the canal.

Manually activated irrigation involves agitation of the irrigant by corono-apical movements of the irrigation needle, stirring movements with small endodontic files and manual push–pull movements with a master gutta percha cone. These allow irrigant in the canal to reach non-instrumented areas (Figure 12.2).

Negative pressure irrigation involves systems such as the EndoVac in which a cannula is placed close to the working length and suction is applied to aspirate away the irrigants. This creates a negative pressure, pulling more irrigant in from the coronal aspect.

Positive pressure irrigation systems deliver the irrigant through a thin needle containing a lateral opening. The fluid is then evacuated through a large needle at the root canal orifice. There is a risk of irrigant extrusion with this technique.

The alternating pressure non-instrumentation technique involves applying positive and negative pressure to the canals via the access cavity. However, there have been reports of severe postoperative pain after this technique and it is now rarely used.

Sonic irrigation devices such as the Endoactivator generate vibrations up to 10 kHz whilst **ultrasonics** vibrate with a frequency above 20 kHz. Passive ultrasonic irrigation either employs special ultrasonic files or uses a normal tip touching a small file that has been placed in the canal. Both sonic and ultrasonic irrigation can cause cavitation and acoustic streaming. Cavitation involves the production of bubbles that can implode to disrupt biofilms. Acoustic streaming is the production of currents in the irrigating solution which can dislodge debris and cause further biofilm disruption. Both sonic and ultrasonic irrigation heat the disinfectant, increasing its efficiency.

Root canal lubricants

Lubricants are used to emulsify debris removed by mechanical instrumentation. They also facilitate the action of the hand and mechanised files to reduce the risk of binding and fracture. Common lubricants include RC-Prep and Glyde. They are based on EDTA and urea peroxide. The latter can react with the NaOCl causing effervescence in the canal but without any risk of causing surgical emphysema.

13 Root canal medicaments

Table 13.1 Indications for endodontic treatment over one and two visits.

Method of management	Indications
Single visit root canal treatment	• Teeth showing irreversible pulpitis or having necrotic pulps with only small periapical areas may have minimal bacterial infection. A permanent coronal seal should be placed as soon as possible to limit further bacterial ingress. • Teeth which require a post-core restoration. Temporary posts provide a very poor seal, and it may be better to complete the root canal treatment in one visit to allow immediate placement of a definitive post, and produce a coronal seal immediately. • Teeth that are at risk of a fracture require a cuspal coverage restoration as soon as possible. Prolonging the treatment over multiple visits extends the period that the tooth is at risk of fracture before a crown can be placed. • Single appointments are more cost effective as the overall treatment time and materials used is less. • Single appointments are often more convenient for patients as they reduce their travelling time, and time off work.
Multiple visit root canal treatment	• If a canal cannot be dried because of persistent pus or bleeding. • Some patients may not be able to tolerate long treatment sessions and would prefer two shorter sessions. • In complex cases, there may be insufficent time to adequately disinfect the root canals in one session. • If the patient has preoperative pain, swelling or a sinus tract, the patient and dentist may benefit in seeing a resolution of signs and symptoms before the canals are obturated. • Teeth that present with large radiographic periapical areas have canals with a greater number and diversity of bacteria. The $Ca(OH)_2$ may be beneficial in reducing this bacterial load as much as possible prior to obturation of the canals.

Box 13.1 Properties of the ideal root canal medicament.

• Broad spectrum antibacterial and antifungal activity
• Must be able to penetrate the dentine tubules
• Biocompatible with the apical tissues
• Ability to control inflammatory exudates and bleeding
• Ability to control pain by reducing the inflammation
• Induce calcific barrier formation in teeth with immature apices
• Limit root resorption
• Must not affect the setting of the temporary filling
• Should be radiopaque
• Must not stain the tooth
• Easy to place and remove
• Inexpensive

Endodontology at a Glance. First Edition. Alix Davies, Federico Foschi and Shanon Patel. © 2019 John Wiley & Sons, Ltd. Published 2019 by John Wiley & Sons, Ltd.
Companion website: www.wiley.com/go/davies/endodontology

Aims of root canal medicaments

If root canal treatment cannot be completed in a single visit, there is the risk that any remaining intracanal bacteria will proliferate between appointments. An intracanal medicament should be placed to eliminate remaining microorganisms. The ideal properties of a root canal medicament are described in Box 13.1.

Available medicaments

Calcium hydroxide

Calcium hydroxide ($Ca(OH)_2$) paste is a slow acting antiseptic that has been shown to significantly decrease the bacterial load within the root canal. It is supplied in a paste form or a powder to which distilled water is added to produce the desired consistency. The paste is then placed into the canal with a file or injected with a syringe. $Ca(OH)_2$ penetrates the dentine tubules and creats a highly alkaline antibacterial environment. Reducing the bacterial count reduces inflammatory exudate and therefore decreases any pain. The alkaline pH created by the $Ca(OH)_2$ also neutralises the acidic inflammatory environment. Calcium hydroxide is biocompatible, non-toxic and non-carcinogenic. However, long-term $Ca(OH)_2$ placement can also reduce the fracture resistance of the tooth. It is inexpensive, radiopaque because of the addition of barium sulfate and does not stain teeth. Removal of $Ca(OH)_2$ is aided by irrigation with EDTA.

$Ca(OH)_2$ can be used to stimulate formation of a hard tissue barrier at the apex of the tooth (apexification). The alkaline environment maintains a bacteria free environment whilst inducing an osteogenic reaction to induce calcific barrier formation. However, its use in this field has been largely superseded by MTA (see Figure 27.4).

Steroid/Antibiotic paste

Odontopaste contains a corticosteroid (triamcinolone) and antibiotic (clindamycin). Its use is advocated in the emergency management of pulpitic procedures. The steroid reduces the inflammation of the pulp to reduce pain. However, it has limited antibacterial effect.

Triple antibiotic paste

This paste contains a mixture of metronidazole, ciprofloxacin and minocycline. Triple antibiotic paste is currently used to eradicate bacteria in pulpal regeneration procedures in immature permanent teeth. However, it can cause severe tooth staining. If triplemix is used, the walls of the coronal third of the root canal and crown should be sealed with dentinal bonding agents to minimise the risk of staining. However, use of antibiotics in this manner can promote antibacterial resistance, and there is a risk of allergic reaction.

Bioactive glass

Bioactive glasses are under development for use as intracanal medicaments. They have been shown to induce dentine mineralisation and exert an antimicrobial effect within the canal by producing a highly alkaline environment. They are non-toxic and biocompatible.

Formaldehyde

Formocresol was extensively used in the past. However, it is highly toxic and has mutagenic and carcinogenic potential. There is no justification for its use in dentistry today.

Should root canal treatment be performed over one or two visits?

There is considerable debate as to whether endodontic treatment should be completed in one or two visits.

The one visit management strategy aims to adequately reduce the bacterial load in one treatment session. It then aims to render the remaining microorganisms harmless by obturating immediately, thus depriving them of nutrients to survive and multiply. The antimicrobial effects of the sealer can also kill residual bacteria. The two visit strategy aims to use an interappointment dressing to further decrease the bacterial load after instrumentation prior to obturation at a second visit.

Laboratory studies comparing the bacterial load of root canals show a decreased number of microorganisms in patients when a calcium hydroxide dressing has been placed. However, this has not translated to improved clinical treatment outcomes. There are no reported differences in postoperative pain or swelling in patients treated in one or multiple visits. Each case should therefore be assessed on an individual basis to determine the best management plan. Indications for one and two visit appointments are described in Table 13.1.

14 Endodontic files

Figure 14.1 Various tapers that may be found on endodontic files.

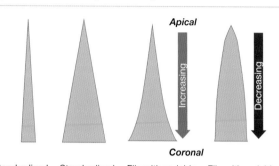

Apical

Increasing

Decreasing

Coronal

Standardised file with a constant narrow taper

Standardised file with a constant wide taper

File with variable increasing taper from apical to coronal direction

File with variable decreasing taper from apical to coronal direction

Figure 14.2 Various files in longitudinal and cross-section.

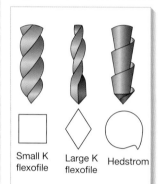

Small K flexofile

Large K flexofile

Hedstrom

Figure 14.3 Rake angle.

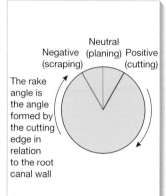

Negative (scraping)

Neutral (planing)

Positive (cutting)

The rake angle is the angle formed by the cutting edge in relation to the root canal wall

Figure 14.4 The balanced force technique.

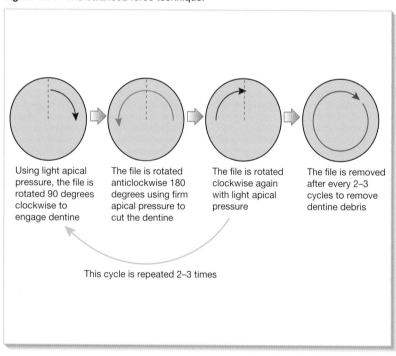

Using light apical pressure, the file is rotated 90 degrees clockwise to engage dentine

The file is rotated anticlockwise 180 degrees using firm apical pressure to cut the dentine

The file is rotated clockwise again with light apical pressure

The file is removed after every 2–3 cycles to remove dentine debris

This cycle is repeated 2–3 times

Figure 14.6 Torsional fatigue.

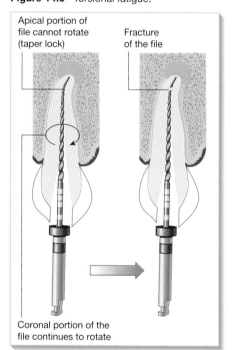

Apical portion of file cannot rotate (taper lock)

Fracture of the file

Coronal portion of the file continues to rotate

Figure 14.5 Cyclical fatigue.

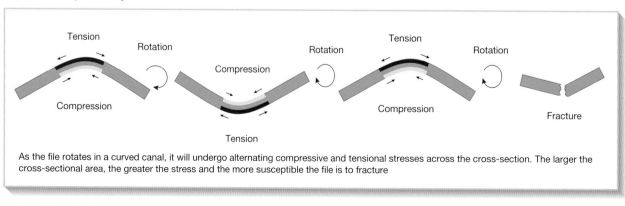

Tension

Rotation

Compression

Compression

Tension

Tension

Rotation

Compression

Rotation

Fracture

As the file rotates in a curved canal, it will undergo alternating compressive and tensional stresses across the cross-section. The larger the cross-sectional area, the greater the stress and the more susceptible the file is to fracture

Endodontology at a Glance. First Endition. Alix Davies, Federico Foschi and Shanon Patel. © 2019 John Wiley & Sons, Ltd. Published 2019 by John Wiley & Sons, Ltd.
Companion website: www.wiley.com/go/davies/endodontology

Hand files

Hand files are available in various apical diameters and tapers. Stainless steel superseded the original carbon steel files to improve the quality of the instruments. Nickel titanium, introduced in the 1990s, demonstrated superior flexibility and resistance to torsional fracture compared with equivalent stainless steel files. It is used to manufacture hand and rotary instruments.

The International Organisation for Standardisation (ISO) and the American National Standards Institute (ANSI) are responsible for defining the dimensions, physical properties and providing quality control for endodontic instruments. Standardisation covers the diameter and taper (Figure 14.1) of each instrument, the graduated increase in size from one instrument to the next and the numbering system for each file.

The most commonly used hand files are variants of K and H files. K files are made of a stainless steel wire that is square or rhomboidal (Figure 14.2) in cross-section and twisted to form flutes. The edge of the flutes provides the cutting surfaces with the space between acting as a reservoir for debris. These may be used with the balanced force or a (gentle) filing technique. The H file is manufactured by milling the file. The most common H file is the Hedström file which has a round surface area with multiple flutes with a positive rake angle (Figure 14.3). It actively cuts in a filing motion and is effective in removing root-filling materials. These files must not be rotated more than 90 degrees otherwise they are likely to fracture.

Rotary files

Rotary files are made of nickel titanium alloys. Their increased flexibility and resistance to fracture allows them to be manufactured with a greater taper than the 2% ISO and to be used in a 360° rotational movement. First generation files were manufactured in 1993 and comprised ProFiles, which had a non-cutting tip and engaged the dentine with a planning action. Generation 2 files (e.g. ProTaper) have an increased cutting action where each file had increasing and decreasing tapers along its length. This allowed more of the instrument to engage the canal wall, this reducing the number of files used. However, these files were still subject to torsional fracture. Third generation files were the product of research focusing on altered manufacturing processes such as heat and surface treatments as well as varying the ratios of the alloys. These were designed to improve flexibility and increase the files' resistance to fracture. These include files such as Profile Vortex, Hyflex and Twisted files. Newer generation files as ProTaper Next have an offset centre of rotation that results in a swaggering movement. This reduces the stresses and risk of fracture. Rotary files have been developed that can be precured prior to use. This is beneficial in severely curved canals and in bypassing ledges.

Reciprocating files

Nickel titanium reciprocating files (generation 4) aim to replicate the balanced force technique (Figure 14.4). Reciprocating files are driven with a reciprocating motor and have unequal angles of rotation. The angle of rotation is lower than the angle of the elastic limit of the instrument, thereby lowering the risk of fracture of the file. Different use with a slightly increased pecking motion should be considered with this type of file because of the reduced threading-in effect compared with rotary files.

Arguments for and against single-use files

In 2007, the UK introduced a policy to make endodontic files single-use. Concerns had been raised over the difficulties in cleaning and sterilising the files. Even after meticulous ultrasonic cleaning and decontamination procedures, organic and inorganic matter was detected on the file surfaces. It was considered that endodontic files could act as a vehicle for transmission of diseases such as variant Creutzfeldt–Jakob disease (vCJD) if they were reused, especially as prion proteins associated with vCJD are resistant to almost every sterilisation method currently used in dental practice. Root canal treatment aims to reduce the bacterial load in root canals or prevent infection in vital inflamed pulps and therefore the use of files that were already contaminated could adversely affect treatment outcomes.

Other reasons for adopting a single-use policy are that files undergoing multiple cycles of clinical instrumentation, cleaning, disinfection and sterilisation show a reduced cutting efficiency and are at an increased risk of instrument fracture. However, the cost implications of using the files once is high.

15 Endodontic armamentarium

Figure 15.1 A selection of available clamps, rubber dam forceps, pliers and frame.

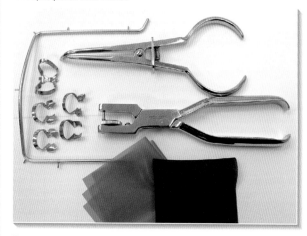

Figure 15.2 Syringes containing endodontic irritants. It is noteworthy that it is not possible to differentiate between the solutions without the use of labels: eucalyptus oil (EO), EDTA and NaOCL.

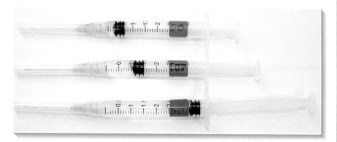

Figure 15.4 EndoRay holder.

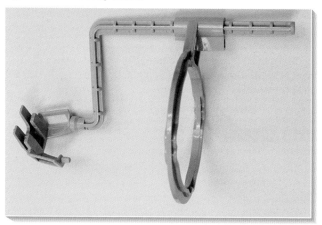

Figure 15.3 An apex locator.

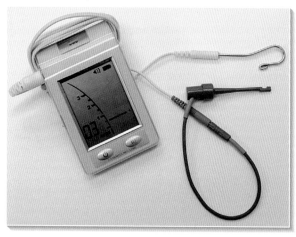

Figure 15.5 Ultrasonic scaler with tips.

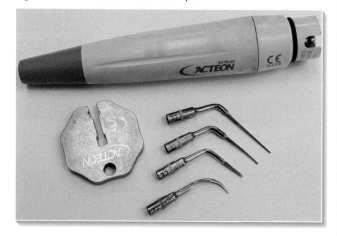

Table 15.1 Comparison of irrigation needle diameters compared with endodontic files.

Irrigation needle gauge size	Diameter of the needle lumen (mm)	Corresponding ISO file (including needle walls)
23	0.6	70
25	0.5	55
27	0.4	45
30	0.3	35

Box 15.1 Advantages of rubber dam use.

- The patient cannot inhale or swallow instruments, irrigating solutions or debris.
- The access cavity and root canals are isolated and cannot be contaminated by bacteria in the saliva, blood or other tissue fluids in the mouth.
- Soft tissues are retracted and therefore protected from burs or heat from the instruments used in warm obturation procedures.
- The rubber dam improves visibility.
- Rubber dam minimises patient conversation and the need for frequent rinsing, therefore makes the procedure more efficient.
- The clinician follows the required standards of care, and is therefore less likely to encounter complications and potential litigation cases.

Endodontology at a Glance. First Edition. Alix Davies, Federico Foschi and Shanon Patel. © 2019 John Wiley & Sons, Ltd. Published 2019 by John Wiley & Sons, Ltd.
Companion website: www.wiley.com/go/davies/endodontology

Rubber dam

Rubber dam use is mandatory to enable root canal treatment to be performed safely and efficiently (Box 15.1).

Rubber dam sheets are available in different thicknesses. Thick sheets are less likely to tear and are more effective at retracting the soft tissues. Thin sheets are easier to place. They also exert less tension through the clamp to the tooth. Rubber dam is also available in a variety of colours, with darker colours providing better contrast with the tooth and the lighter colours providing greater illumination of the operating field. Latex and latex free sheets are available.

Rubber dam clamps anchor the dam to the most posterior tooth that requires isolation. They are composed of stainless steel and comprise two jaws connected by a bow. Winged clamps additionally show a winged extension to the jaws which allows the rubber dam and the clamp to be placed at the same time. The wing enhances soft tissue retraction. A variety of clamps are available to fit various anatomical configurations of all tooth types. Rubber dam frames are required to retract and stabilise the rubber dam. A rubber dam punch and forceps are also required (Figure 15.1). In anterior teeth, wedjets can be used to stabilise the dam instead of clamps.

Irrigating syringes and needles

A variety of irrigating needle diameters are available. Side venting needles should be used to allow backflow of irrigant and minimise extrusion into the periapical spaces (see Chapter 22). Syringes should be labelled showing their contents (Figure 15.2); a Luer lock design is preferable to allow easy unscrewing of the needle to replenish the syringe without risk of unintentional detaching of the needle. Appropriate gauge should be selected to reach as close as possible to the working length, without risking extrusion (Table 15.1).

Apex locators

The ideal preparation and obturation point for root canals is the apical constriction, as this is where the pulp tissue converges with the periodontal ligament (see Chapter 11). An estimate of the root canal length can be obtained from radiographs, tactile sensation and the presence of bleeding on paper points. However, these methods have limited accuracy.

An electronic apex locator (Figure 15.3) is a device that measures the position of the apical foramen. This allows the operator to determine the working length of the root canal. In addition to determining the apical foramen position, apex locators can also be used to assess the presence and position of root fractures and perforations.

Newer generation apex locators measure the impedence (the ratio of voltage to current in an alternating current circuit) or the ratio of impedences to determine the apical foramen position. This follows the principle that two or more electrical alternating currents with different wave frequencies have different impedances that can be measured and compared as a ratio, even when there is fluid in the canal. This allows accurate measurements to be made, even in 'wet' canals. The latest generation apex locators can compare the impedence measurements with values recorded on a database. This allows the distance between the file and the apex to be calculated. Previous generations of apex locator only provided accurate information when the file was at the apical foramen.

Apex locator results need to be confirmed by taking measurements with radiographs as they can still provide inaccurate readings, especially if excess irrigant or inflammatory exudate is present. Short circuiting can occur if the file with the electrode contacts metallic restorations or instruments in other canals. If isolation is poor, saliva can conduct the current to the gingival tissues, again producing a false reading. The apex locator is most accurate when the file touches the canal walls. Wide canals with immature apical foramina therefore produce less reliable readings. The largest possible passive file should be used for this reason.

Film holders

Film holders are essential when using the paralleling technique as they reduce the risk of distortion and cone cutting (see Chapter 7). They allow more reproducible radiograph angulations. When taking radiographs with endodontic files or gutta percha points in situ, specialised holders such as the XCP and EndoRay holders (Figure 15.4) aid alignment by fitting over clamps and files.

Ultrasonics

Ultrasonics vibrate at a frequency above 20 Hz. This vibration is produced either by magnetostrictive units or piezoelectric units. Piezoelectric units are preferential in endodontics. They contain a crystal that changes shape when current is applied. This change is converted into mechanical oscillation. The oscillation is a piston movement rather than lateral movement and therefore allows finer control of the handpiece and minimises excessive dentine removal. The units can produce frequencies of up to 40 Hz. Varying ultrasonic tips can be attached to the handpiece (Figure 15.5). This tips have differing roles: locating calicified canals, removing posts and separated instruments, activating irrigant (see Chapter 12) and condensation of root filling materials.

16 Obturation

Figure 16.1 Stages in cold lateral condensation. (a) A gutta percha point corresponding to the master file size is tried into the prepared canal to the working length. (b) The gutta percha point is coated in sealer and placed back in the canal. A finger spreader is inserted 1 mm short of the working length. This compacts the gutta percha and provides space for the accessory point. (c) The finger spreader is removed and an accessory point is coated in sealer and placed in the space that has been created. (d) The finger spreader is inserted 2–3 mm short of the working length. (e) The finger spreader is removed and an accessory point is coated in sealer and placed in the space that has been created. (f) The finger spreader inserted 4–5 mm short of the working length. (g) The process continues with the finger spreader 1 mm shorter each time. (h) The excess filling material can be seared off with a heated plugger.

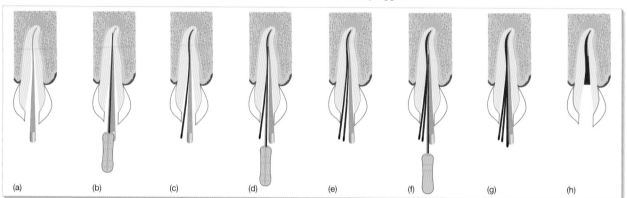

(a)   (b)   (c)   (d)   (e)   (f)   (g)   (h)

Figure 16.2 Stages of warm vertical compaction. (a) A gutta percha point of the correct apical gauge corresponding to the master file size is tried into the prepared canal to the working length. A radiograph is taken to confirm the correct position and adjustments are made if required. (b) The heated plugger tip is tried into the canal to ensure that it can be placed to within 5mm of the working length. (c) The gutta percha is coated in sealer and placed in the root canal. This is then seared off using an electrically heated plugger. (d) A plugger is used to compact the apical gutta percha. (e) The remaining canal wall is coated in sealer prior to backfilling the canal with heated, softened gutta percha. (f) A plugger is used to compact the coronal gutta percha.

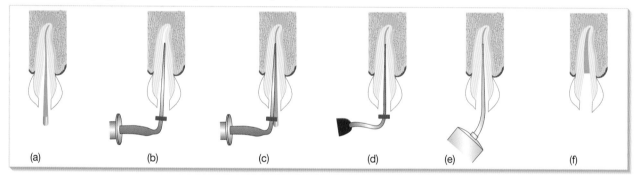

(a)   (b)   (c)   (d)   (e)   (f)

Box 16.1 The ideal properties of a root filling material.

- Easy manipulation and good working time
- Dimensionally stable with no shrinkage or dissolution over time
- Ability to flow to fill the complex internal anatomy of the tooth and seal the canal apically and laterally
- Adhesive to dentine
- Not irritating to the periapical tissues
- Non-porous
- Non-corrosive and must not oxidise in the presence of moisture
- Antibacterial
- Radiopaque and easily identifiable on radiography
- Not cause tooth discoloration
- Sterile
- Easy to remove by being soluble in a common solvent
- Inexpensive

Box 16.2 Components of gutta percha cones.

• Gutta percha	20%
• Zinc oxide (filler)	65%
• Heavy metal salts (radiopacifier)	10%
• Waxes and resins (plasticisers)	5%

Box 16.3 Properties of an ideal root canal sealer.

- Good working time
- Soluble in common solvent if root filling removal is required
- Radiopaque
- Good adhesive and cohesive strength
- No shrinkage on setting
- No staining of the tooth structure
- Produces a completely airtight seal
- Bactericidal
- Insoluble in tissue fluids
- Non-irritant, not toxic or mutagenic
- No effect on the set of the permanent coronal filling

Endodontology at a Glance. First Edition. Alix Davies, Federico Foschi and Shanon Patel. © 2019 John Wiley & Sons, Ltd. Published 2019 by John Wiley & Sons, Ltd.
Companion website: www.wiley.com/go/davies/endodontology

Obturation of root canals

Obturation aims to fill the root canal space and, in doing so, eliminate all portals of exit between the canal and the periodontal ligament. The root filling can also prevent bacteria re-entering the canal via percolation from the apical tissues. Bactericidal effects of the sealer kill or prevent regrowth of any remaining microorganisms. The filling material should entomb any microorganisms that are not eradicated during chemodebridement to prevent their egress to the periodontal ligament. If the coronal seal is lost because of caries, fracture of a restoration or the tooth, the root filling also provides an additional barrier to limit the passage of bacteria through the root canal. The ideal properties of a root filling material are described in Box 16.1.

Root filling materials

Gutta percha is the most commonly placed root filling materials. Root canals were previously filled with various resins (e.g. Russian red) and silver points. However, these produce a poor seal and can be challenging to remove, so they are now considered below the standard of care required. In certain cases (e.g. immature root development), bioceramic materials (e.g. MTA, Biodentine) may be used.

Gutta percha

Gutta percha points are composed predominantly of zinc oxide and gutta percha (Box 16.2). Gutta percha is a trans isomer of polyisoprene. It is radiopaque and easily identifiable on radiographs. Gutta percha is usually pink and therefore can 'show through' and cause some discoloration if the remaining tooth tissue is very thin. This problem can be overcome by ensuring that the filling is seared off at the neck of the tooth. Although gutta percha points cannot be heat sterilised, they can be disinfected prior to use by soaking in a solution of 5.25% NaOCl for 1 minute.

Gutta percha oxidises and can become brittle over time on exposure to light. It exists in solid form at room temperature, still maintaining a good compactability which can be utilised for the cold lateral condensation technique. This technique allows for controlled placement of gutta percha in the root canal. The final filling is composed of a large number of gutta percha cones (master and accessories points) that are tightly pressed together and adhere via frictional grip and the presence of the sealer (Figure 16.1). This technique is easy to learn and is inexpensive.

Thermoplasticised gutta percha involves warming the gutta percha to above 65°C where it exists in a pliable form and flows more easily. It can be used it many different applications.

Warm vertical compaction

The stages of warm vertical condensation are shown in Figure 16.2. Various heating systems are available to use. This technique is quick and produces well-filled canals with minimal voids. The pressure also allows irregularities such as resorption defects and accessory canals to be filled. There is less control of overfill and therefore care must be taken to ensure the canal has been apically gauged and a gutta percha point of the correct apical size is chosen. The canal must also be tapered to resist apical migration of the gutta percha point. The equipment for warm vertical condensation is relatively expensive.

Warm lateral compaction

This technique involves the placement of a master cone prior to using a heated spreader to provide space for accessory points. It decreases the pressure placed on the tooth and the risk of extrusion of the root filling material.

Carrier-based gutta percha

This method uses a solid carrier coated in gutta percha. The carrier and gutta percha are heated in a controlled fashion before being placed in the canal to the working length. The rigid core allows for speedy placement. However, length control is difficult and excessive extrusion may be seen. The sealer cannot be coated on the gutta percha point but rather applied to the root canal walls prior to obturation. In addition, the apical gutta percha can be stripped so that the core is exposed and acts as the obturator. This does not create a good seal and can lead to potential microbial leakage. Other disadvantages of carrier-based obturation include difficulty in removing the carrier for retreatments, and difficulty in placing posts. The ovens for heating the carrier-based systems and the points are also expensive.

Bioceramic cements

Bioceramic materals (e.g. MTA and Biodentine) can also be used as a conventional root filling, especially for patients with large open apices caused by incomplete root development or resorption.

Single cone

The development of an effective single cone technique is still in its infancy. The use of bioceramic sealers in conjunction with greater taper gutta percha point have been advocated. Generous coating with sealer of a cone matching the taper and gauge of the master greater taper file has been suggested. However, the anatomy of certain canals (e.g. palatal root of maxillary molars and distal root of mandibular molar) can lead to discrepancies and voids.

Root canal sealers

The sealer aims to fill the space between the filling material and the dentine. Ideal properties of root canal sealers are shown in Box 16.3. A variety of sealers of different materials are available, including the following:
- Calcium hydroxide based (Sealapex, RealSeal, Apexit)
- Zinc oxide eugenol based (Tubliseal, Roth's pulp canal sealer)
- Glass ionomer based (Ketac-Endo)
- Resin sealers (AH26, AH Plus, Epiphany, EndoREZ)
- Silicone sealers (RoekoSeal, GuttaFlow)
- Bioceramic sealers (BioRoot, EndoSequence BC).

17 Root canal retreatment

Figure 17.1 Braiding technique for Hedström files for removing silver points. (a) Cement around silver point gently removed with ultrasonics and solvent. (b) Two or three Hedström files are braided around the silver point. (c) The Hedström files are twisted around to engage the silver point. (d) Files are steadily pulled coronally to remove the silver point.

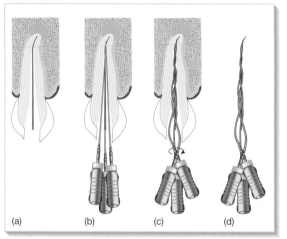

(a)   (b)   (c)   (d)

Figure 17.2 (a) Components of the instrument removal system (i) screw and (ii) microtube. The screw fits into the microtube (iii) to engage with the file. (b) Canal with retained file. (c) Microtube placed into canal with bevel towards outer edge of the curve. (d) Screw introduced into microtube. It is rotated anticlockwise until it engages with the file and displaces it out of the side opening. (e) Microtube with retrieved fractured file.

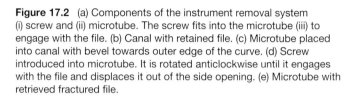
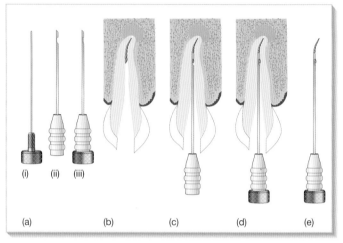

(i) (ii) (iii)

(a)   (b)   (c)   (d)   (e)

Table 17.1 Indications and contraindications to retreatment.

Indications for root canal retreatment	Contraindications for root canal retreatment
Persistent pain or pain that develops after a period of time following root canal treatment	Asymptomatic teeth with no evidence of apical pathology despite a poor root treatment, providing no complex treatment is planned for the tooth
Development of a new swelling or sinus tract, or failure of a sinus tract to resolve after treatment	Presence of ledges, perforations or fractured instruments that are unlikely to be successfully managed non-surgically. A surgical approach may be preferred in these cases
Radiographic evidence of an enlarging periapical area	Root canal treatment has already been performed to a good standard, and would be difficult to improve. A surgical approach may be more beneficial
Planning of a cuspal coverage restoration on a tooth with a periapical area and/or a tooth that has an inadequate root canal treatment	Teeth that are unrestorable because of extensive caries, or that have cracks or root fractures
Planning of a cuspal coverage restoration on a tooth where the existing root canal filling is exposed to the oral environment (because of caries or restoration fracture) for an extended period of time	

Table 17.2 Factors affecting prognosis of perforations.

Location of the perforation	A coronal perforation is easier to repair because of improved access. This will have a good prognosis providing the remainder of the canal can still be fully instrumented and disinfected. In cases where the canal cannot be instrumented beyond the perforation, the more apical the perforation, the better the prognosis, as more of the canal has been disinfected
Time delay prior to perforation repair	Immediate repair is preferable as any delay may allow breakdown of the periodontium and cause a perio-endo lesion which is difficult to manage
Ability to seal the perforation defect	A good seal is critical to prevent egress of microorganisms
Previous contamination of the canal	If the canal is contaminated with microorganisms, the prognosis is lower, especially if the canal cannot be instrumented beyond the point of the perforation

Endodontology at a Glance. First Edition. Alix Davies, Federico Foschi and Shanon Patel. © 2019 John Wiley & Sons, Ltd. Published 2019 by John Wiley & Sons, Ltd.
Companion website: www.wiley.com/go/davies/endodontology

Root canal retreatment is more challenging than primary endodontic treatment. Indications and contraindications for retreatment are shown in Table 17.1. The chances of success are usually lower than for primary treatment.

Retreatment requires re-establishment of coronal access, removing all coronal restorations (see Chapter 10). Posts must be removed along with the existing root filling material and if possible, any fractured instruments. Ideally, canals should be instrumented and disinfected to the apical constriction. This involves negotiation of ledges or blockages and identification and disinfection of additional previously missed canals.

Post removal

The coronal aspect should be exposed. Ultrasonic tips are then used with copious irrigation to disrupt the cement lute at the interface of the tooth and the post. Post removal kits may be used on posts which are broken and embedded in the root canal. Fibre posts can be removed by drilling through the centre of the post using specialised post removal drills. This softens the matrix that binds the post fibres, allowing their removal.

Removal of root fillings

A variety of root fillings can require removal. Gutta percha may have been used in conjuction with a carrier. Historical obturation materials include silver points and resin paste fillers.

Gutta percha can be removed from the coronal portion of the canal with a heated plugger or Gates Glidden burs. It can often be removed from the apical third by mechanical instrumentation alone, especially if the filling was poorly condensed. However, in cases where the filling was well condensed, a solvent such as chloroform or eucalyptus oil can be used to soften the material. Retreatment files can also help. Resilon is removed in the same way as gutta percha. However, the resin sealer often remains and can be removed with specialised resin solvents.

Retreatment of patients with carrier-based fillings are more difficult as the carrier has often been wedged into an incompletely prepared canal. A solvent is used to soften the gutta percha and create space around the carrier. Ultrasonics can also be used for this purpose. Stieglitz forceps can then be used to engage with and extract the carrier. Hedström files may also be used to engage with the carriers and assist with their removal.

Silver points are often embedded in the filling that forms the core of the tooth. The filling must be removed, aiming to keep the silver point intact. The access cavity should then be flooded with a solvent to dissolve any cement. If the point is tightly held in place, ultrasonics can be used to gently loosen the cement around the point, prior to grasping and removing it with Stieglitz forceps. A gentle continuous force should be applied to increase the chance of removing the point intact. Hedström files can also be used to remove the point using the braiding technique (Figure 17.1).

Removal of paste fillers is unpredictable. Solvents such as chloroform and eucalyptus oil are often ineffective and a resin solvent is required. Ultrasonic files can assist with removal of the coronal paste. Often, the apical portions are inadequately filled and, once accessed, can be successfully instrumented and disinfected.

Removal of fractured instruments

Instrument fracture is a complication of root canal treatment that can prevent disinfection of the portion of the canal apical to it. The fractured instrument is usually a hand or rotary file but can also be part of a Gates Glidden drill or spiral paste filler.

If the fractured instrument is in the coronal portion of the canal, or there is straight line access to it, removal is often possible. In some cases, the instrument can be grasped with a haemostat or Stieglitz forceps. Ultrasonic tips on low power settings can be used to loosen a file that has separated deeper in the canal. Various extractor systems are available, most commonly using a microtube that is inserted over the instrument. This may be used in conjunction with adhesive to bond the tube to the file, or with a wedge (wire, screw or Hedström file) to bind to the instrument and facilitate its removal (Figure 17.2).

Negotiation of ledges and blockages

After the root filling materials have been removed, it may still not be possible to instrument to the apical constriction if the canal has been blocked or ledged. It is then necessary to enlarge the coronal portion of the canal in conjunction with copious irrigation. The canal should then be gently probed with a file of size 8 or 10 to scout for 'sticky' spots that may be the entrance to the canal. Gentle 'pecking' at this point allows advancement of the file and opens up the canal to enable disinfection. A radiograph should be taken to confirm progress is in the right direction to minimise the risk of perforation. If a ledge is encountered, a fine file should be precurved in an attempt to bypass it and recapture the original pathway. If this is successful, a short push–pull technique should be applied, keeping the file apical to the ledge. This enlarges it enough to allow a sequentially larger file to bypass the ledge until the ledge can be blended in with the canal. If this is not possible, the patient should be advised of the guarded prognosis and the tooth should be monitored. Apical surgery may become necessary in the future.

Perforation repair

Root perforations can occur iatrogenically during root canal treatment or during post placement. Various factors affect the prognosis of perforations (Table 17.2). Non-surgical perforation repair involves location and instrumentation of the canals beyond the perforation and irrigation of the defect with sterile saline. Gutta percha cones should be placed in the canal to prevent blocking it beyond the perforation. MTA or Biodentine should then be placed in the defect and allowed to set prior to final preparation and obturation of the root canal system.

18 Surgical endodontic treatment

Figure 18.1 (a) Ultrasonic tips used for microsurgical canal preparation (b) Pritchard Periosteal elevator, (c) micromirror and (d) microedges.

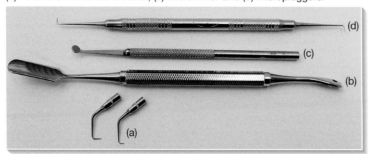

Box 18.1 Contraindications to root end surgery.

- Poor periodontal support
- Unfavourable crown to root ratio
- Poor root canal filling that can be improved
- Poor coronal seal (caries or poorly placed restorations)
- Difficult access (upper palatal roots, lower molar roots)
- Risk of damage to structures such as the inferior dental nerve, mental nerve or maxillary sinus
- Patients with bleeding disorders, undergoing radiotherapy or taking bisphosphonates should avoid treatment if possible

Figure 18.2 (a) Preoperative periapical showing a lesion on the mesial root. (b) Radiograph showing the mesial root resection and MTA root end filling. (c) Radiographic review 1 year later shows resolution of the lesion.

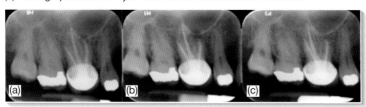

Box 18.2 Properties of an ideal root end filling material.

- Non-toxic and non-carcinogenic
- Biocompatible with the host tissues
- Insoluble in tissue fluids
- Dimensionally stable over time
- Easy to use
- Non-staining
- Radiopaque
- Produces a good seal

Table 18.1 Advantages and disadvantages of various flap designs.

Horizontal incision	Description		Advantages	Disadvantages
Limited mucoperiosteal flaps				
Semilunar incision	Horizontal incision in the alveolar mucosa		Minimises recession of the gingivae Fast procedure	Poor access to the surgical field Difficult to reapproximate the margins and extensive scarring can occur
Submarginal incision	Flap is raised within the gingiva leaving 4 mm of attached gingivae present at the margin		Crown margins are completely untouched and recession is minimised Can be used in cases where concurrent surgical and non-surgical endodontic procedures are being performed as the incisions will not interfere with rubber dam placement	If too little attached gingivae is left behind, the entire region can under go necrosis resulting in very poor aesthetics The incision line may be over the defect and closure will not be on healthy bone There is the potential for scarring Root fractures and periodontal defects can be missed
Full mucoperiosteal flaps				
Papillary-based incision	Papilla is excluded in the incision		Reduces postoperative gingival recession	Harder to perform than other techniques
Sulcular full thickness flap	Entire thickness of gingivae including papilla is included in design		Easy to perform Good visualisation of root and bone	Unpredictable gingival shrinkage and recession

Endodontology at a Glance. First Edition. Alix Davies, Federico Foschi and Shanon Patel. © 2019 John Wiley & Sons, Ltd. Published 2019 by John Wiley & Sons, Ltd.
Companion website: www.wiley.com/go/davies/endodontology

Indications for root end surgery

Root end surgery aims to gain access to and remove the apex of the root. This facilitates removal of the bulk of bacteria that remain when conventional root canal treatment has been unsuccessful. A root end filling seals the canal to prevent recontamination.

Root end surgery is indicated when there is persistent periapical inflammation after root canal treatment or retreatment has been attempted. An additional conventional approach is unlikely to work because:

• Non-surgical approach is impaired because of a previously ledged or blocked canal, or a fractured instrument which cannot be negotiated.
• The lesion persists despite placement of a good quality endodontic treatment. This indicates resiliant bacteria, extraradicular biofilms or a cyst.
• Dismantling the tooth by conventional methods can render the tooth unrestorable. This may be the case in heavily restored teeth including those with posts. However, most posts can be removed successfully without fracture.
• Perforation repair can require a surgical approach.

The cost implications of removal of restorations for retreatment and replacement of those restorations (such as a bridge) may be too high, and the patient may therefore opt for root end surgery in some cases where non-surgical retreatment is possible.

Contraindications to root end surgery are shown in Box 18.1.

Preoperative considerations

Informed consent must be obtained prior to treatment and they should be advised to take non-steroidal anti-inflammatory drug (NSAIDs) before the procedure, providing there are no medical contraindications,. Local anaesthetic with a vasoconstrictor should be used to aid haemostasis and improve visualisation of the surgical field. Buccal and palatal infiltrations should be extended beyond the anticipated flap margins. A preoperative chlorhexidine rinse can be used providing the patient has no reported allergy.

Flap design and care

Retraction of a soft tissue flap is necessary to provide adequate access to the apical lesion. The flap must be designed to avoid damaging structures including the mental nerve, frenal and muscle attachments.

Flap elevation requires a horizontal incision with one or two vertical relieving incisions. Horizontal incisions include semilunar, submarginal, papillary-based incisions and full thickness sulcular incisions (Table 18.1).

The relieving incision(s) should be made on healthy bone and run as vertically as possible. This minimises scarring and bleeding whilst maintaining good perfusion to the flap. The papilla, muscle and frenal attachments must be included or excluded in the flap, not cut through. If the incision is made to the tooth, it should meet at right angles to prevent creating a fine friable wedge of soft tissue that can tear easily. During the procedure, the flap must remain hydrated and be retracted adequately to prevent crushing or tearing of the tissues.

Osteotomy

Once the flap has been retracted, it may be possible to visualise the lesion if the cortical plate has been perforated. Otherwise, measuring the root length on the radiograph and transferring this measurement to the surgical site aids determination of the position of the lesion. The overlying bone must be removed to allow adequate access to aid removal of the periapical inflammatory tissue. This is performed most effectively with a rear venting microsurgical handpiece. Adequate irrigation is necessary to prevent excessive heat generation and subsequent bone necrosis.

Root end resection and preparation

Most apical deltas and additional accessory or lateral canals exist in the apical 3 mm of the root, therefore removal of this portion is indicated. However, a greater length of root may need to be removed if ledges, perforations or fractured files are present coronally. Bevelling the root is not recommended as this would expose the dentine tubules allowing microorganism leakage. The root tip should instead be resected perpendicularly to the long axis of the tooth. The resected end should be inspected under magnification to check for cracks.

Sharp curettes can be used to remove the granulation tissue. This should be sent for histopathological assessment.

The root canal should then be prepared to a depth of at least 3 mm. Ultrasonic tips are now recommended to perform the canal preparation (Figure 18.1). They are easier to orientate and produce a deeper and more retentive preparation. Any isthmi should be included in the preparation.

Root end fillings

The ideal properties of a root end filling material are described in Box 18.2. These characteristics were not all present in pre-existing root filling materials such as amalgam, composite, glass ionomers and zinc oxide eugenol preparations. Therefore MTA was developed in the 1990s.

The main constituents of MTA are tricalcium silicate, tricalcium aluminate, calcium silicate and tetra calcium aluminoferrite. Bismuth oxide is also included for radiopacity. White and grey MTA are available, with the former containing lower amounts of iron, aluminium and magnesium. When MTA is mixed with sterile water, it develops a high pH that is antibacterial. Setting times vary from 15 minutes to 4 hours depending on the MTA type used. It expands on setting which helps produce a good seal. It is not toxic or mutagenic and once set is insoluble. MTA also enhances hard tissue formation. It can be placed using a carrier and microplugger. Micromirrors are also available to ensure the filling is well adapted to the cavity walls (Figure 18.1).

Sutures

The soft tissue flap must be repositioned and compressed. Non-absorbable monofilament sutures are recommended to reattach the flap as they cause less plaque build-up, therefore less inflammation.

Review

Suture removal is recommended after 4 days. Additional clinical reviews are necessary to confirm soft tissue healing. A radiographic review is recommended at least 6 months after the surgery (Figure 18.2). However, bony healing, especially of the cortical plates, may take over a year and extended reviews may be required.

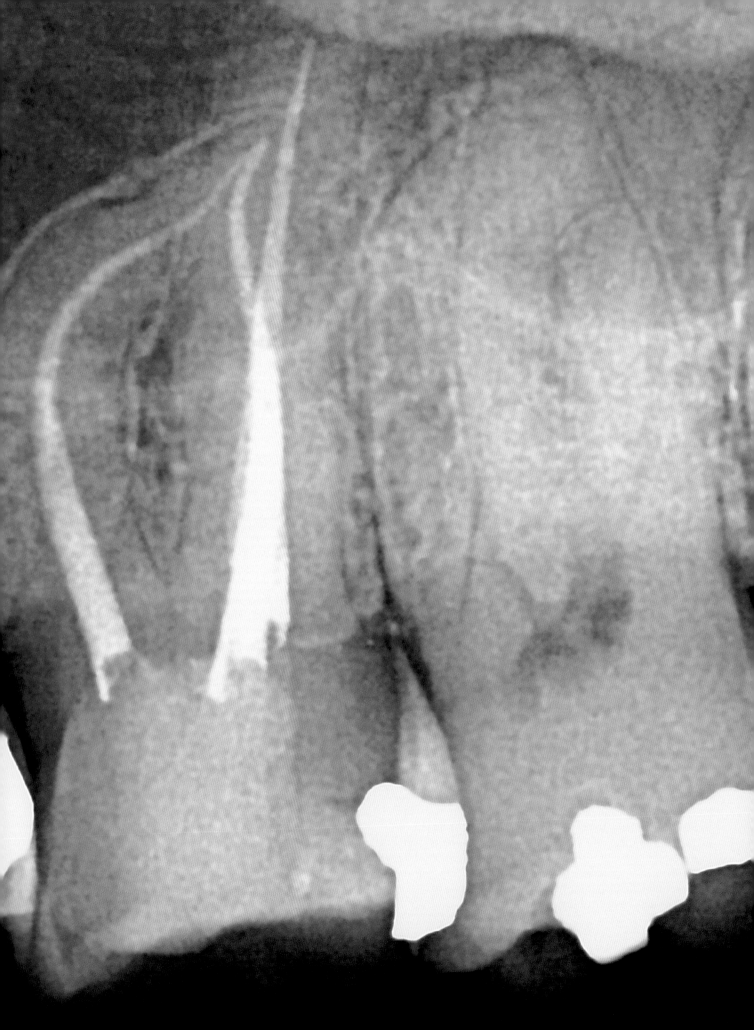

Pain and pain management

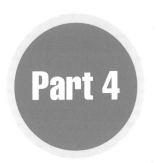

Part 4

Chapters

19 Odontogenic and non-odontogenic pain

Figure 19.1 Many primary afferent neurones converge on to one secondary afferent neurone, and many secondary afferent neurones converge on to one tertiary afferent neurone. Pain from a nociceptor from the mandibular branch of the trigeminal can therefore not only cause referred pain elsewhere along this branch (i.e. to a lower molar), but also to the maxillary branch.

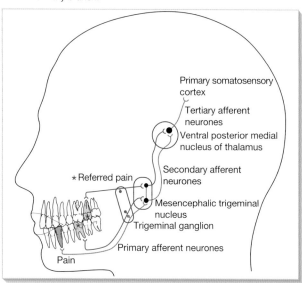

Figure 19.2 This patient presented complaining of prolonged pain to hot and cold around the teeth on the right side. (a) Radiographs were taken and the LR5 was considered to be the cause of the problem. This tooth was accessed and a pulp dressing placed. However, the pain remained unchanged and she was subsequently referred for an opinion as to the cause. Thorough examination with an additional radiograph (b) showing the entire UR8 demonstrated deep caries on the distal aspect of it. Extraction of this has removed the patient's pain. However, failure to make the correct diagnosis in the first instance has resulted in an unnecessary root canal treatment on the LR5.

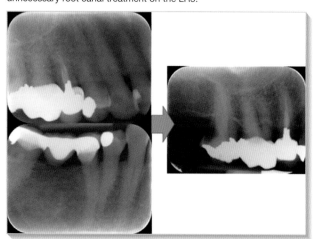

Figure 19.3 Tongue indentations (a) and linea alba (b) on cheek.

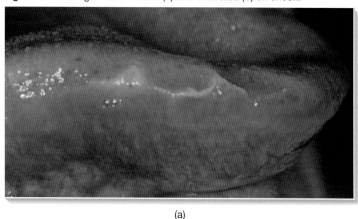

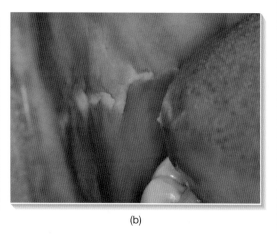

(a)   (b)

Table 19.1 Causes and features of odontogenic and non-odontogenic pain.

Odontogenic causes	Localisation	Onset	Duration	Character
Reversible or irreversible pulpitis	May be difficult to localise	Fast	Variable depending on severity	Throbbing
Dentine hypersensitivity	Localised	Instantaneous	Instantaneous	Sharp sensitivity
Acute apical periodontitis	Localised	Fast	Constant	Extreme tenderness
Acute apical abscess	Localised	Fast	Constant	Extreme tenderness
Acute periodontal abscess	Localised	Fast	Constant	Extreme tenderness
Pericoronitis	Localised	Fast	Constant	Extreme tenderness
Alveolar osteitis	Localised	Fast	Constant	Extreme tenderness
Non-odontogenic causes				
Musculoskeletal	Diffuse	Slow	Constant	Dull
Neurovascular pain	Diffuse	Variable	Intermittent	Throbbing, pulsatile
Neuropathic pain	Localised	Variable	Variable – often short bursts of pain	Shocking, burning
Pain of purely psychological origin	Variable	Variable	Often present constantly	Variable
Pain associated with a pathological process	Diffuse	Slow	Constant	Dull

Endodontology at a Glance. First Edition. Alix Davies, Federico Foschi and Shanon Patel. © 2019 John Wiley & Sons, Ltd. Published 2019 by John Wiley & Sons, Ltd.
Companion website: www.wiley.com/go/davies/endodontology

Pain is as an unpleasant sensory or emotional experience that can be associated with actual or potential tissue damage. Pain reported from the oral structures is either odontogenic (related to the tooth) or non-odontogenic (not of dental origin) (Table 19.1). A detailed pain history is invaluable in formulating a differential diagnosis. A medical history should also be taken as systemic diseases such as rheumatoid arthritis, chronic nerve problems or migraines can be associated with non-odontogenic pain. Current medications should also be documented. A thorough examination is required before selecting appropriate special tests to determine the origin and cause. If there is doubt as to the diagnosis, or it appears to be non-odontogenic, the patient should be referred to the appropriate secondary care department.

Pain history

Details that must be established in the pain history include the following.

Localisation

The patient should be asked where they feel pain. They may be able to localise the offending tooth if the periodontal tissues are inflamed. However, pain of purely pulpal origin can be poorly localised. Non-odontogenic pain can be localised or diffuse and superficial or deep. Easily localised superficial pain tends to be neuropathic whilst musculoskeletal pain is felt more deeply and is harder to localise. Visceral pain is often deep and diffuse.

Referred pain is the perception of pain at a different location to the actual source of the pain (Figure 19.1). This can complicate the diagnosis and increase the risk of 'treating' the wrong tooth (Figure 19.2). Pain of non-odontogenic origin can be referred to the teeth and pain of odontogenic origin can be referred to other areas of the head and neck. Symptoms are usually localised within the same dermatome and tend to occur closer to the nerve origin than the actual source of the pain (e.g. premolar pain is more likely to be referred to a molar tooth than an incisor).

Pain that projects distally along a nerve branch suggests a neuropathic origin. Pain crossing the midline can indicate psychogenic pain whilst maxillary pain that changes position as the patient's posture alters can indicate sinus inflammation.

Onset

The patient should be asked when the pain started and whether anything triggered it. They may recall biting hard on something, losing a filling or having recent dental treatment. These suggest an odontogenic cause but care must be taken not to jump to conclusions. Odontogenic pain usually has a quicker onset than non-odontogenic pain.

Character

Establishment of the quality and severity of the pain is an important part of the pain history. Muscular pain usually manifests as a dull ache. Neurogenic pain is characterised by a burning sensation. Pain of vascular origin (i.e. headache) is often throbbing and pulsating. Odontogenic pain can vary from occasional sensitivity or tenderness to touch to a constant throbbing.

Initiation and relief of pain

Odontogenic pain is usually stimulated by thermal changes, or biting on the affected tooth. Whilst cold can elicit the symptoms, conversely it sometimes relieves pulpitic pain. Non-odontogenic pain such as trigeminal neuralgia can have trigger points but others are less specific. It is important to assess alleviating factors. If the cause of the pain is inflammatory in origin, NSAIDs would be expected to provide some relief. Enquiries should be made into additional accompanying signs or symptoms. Swelling is typical of an infective or inflammatory cause whilst paraesthesia indicates a neuropathy. Nausea, dizziness or abnormal motor function indicates systemic, metabolic or intracranial abnormalities.

Assessment

A thorough extraoral examination must be completed to assess asymmetry, lymphadenopathy or swelling. If pain is considered to be of muscular origin, then the muscles should be palpated to determine any tenderness.

Intraoral examination involves the assessment of the soft tissues for swellings, lesions and sinus tracts. Signs of cheek biting (linea alba) and tongue indentations are indicators of parafunctional activity (Figure 19.3). Teeth should be examined for mobility, wear, decay, large restorations and deep probing depths. They should also be apically and laterally percussed. Palpation in the sulcus at a position overlying the root apices provides some information about the inflammatory state of the periapical tissues. Whilst the intraoral examination mainly assists in the diagnosis of odontogenic problems, a lack of findings can indicate a non-odontogenic cause.

Special tests

Special tests are used for differential diagnosis. They involve the use of hot and cold stimulation to replicate the patient's pain, vitality testing and use of a tooth slooth. Local anaesthetic can also be used to localise the region of the pain (see Chapter 5).

Conventional dental radiographs can provide information about periodontal support, the restorative status of the teeth, periapical pathology and root fractures (see Chapter 7). More specialised radiographic images may be used for non-odontogenic conditions to assess central nervous system lesions (CT scans), salivary glands (sialography), temporomandibular joints (dental panoramic tomography (DTP) and arthography) and blood vessels (angiography). However, these specialised radiographic investigations would usually be requested by oral and maxillofacial, ENT and/or oral medicine specialists.

20 Local anaesthesia in endodontics

Table 20.1 Features of Aδ and C fibres.

	Aδ	**C**
Stimuli	Pressure and thermal stimuli	Pressure, thermal and chemical stimuli
Sensation	Sharp, pricking sensation	Dull aching pain
Presence of a myelin sheath	Yes	No
Diameter (μm)	1–5	0.2–1.5
Conduction speed (m/s)	5–40	0.5–2.0

Table 20.2 Commonly available local anaesthetics that are used in dentistry.

Anaesthetic agent	Commercial name	Manufacturer	Ampoule size	Vasoconstrictor	Latex free
Lidocaine 2%	Xylocaine	Dentsply	2.2	Adrenaline 1 : 80 000	Yes
	Lignospan Special	Septodont	1.8 or 2.2	Adrenaline 1 : 80 000	Yes
	Lignokent	Kent Express	2.2	Adrenaline 1 : 80 000	Yes
Articaine 4%	Septanest 1 : 100 000	Septodont	2.2	Adrenaline 1 : 100 000	Yes
	Septanest 1 : 200 000	Septodont	2.2	Adrenaline 1 : 200 000	Yes
	Artikent	Kent Express	2.2	Adrenaline 1 : 100 000	Yes
Prilocaine 3%	Citanest 3%	Dentsply	2.2	Felypressin 0.03 IU/mL	Yes
Mepivicaine 2%	Scandonest 2% Special	Septodont	2.2	Adrenaline 1 : 100 000	Yes
Mepivicaine 3%	Scandonest 3% plain	Septodont	2.2	None	Yes

Endodontology at a Glance. First Edition. Alix Davies, Federico Foschi and Shanon Patel. © 2019 John Wiley & Sons, Ltd. Published 2019 by John Wiley & Sons, Ltd.
Companion website: www.wiley.com/go/davies/endodontology

The trigeminal nerve comprises three major branches that are predominantly sensory for the orofacial tissues. The maxillary and mandibular branches supply sensation to their respective arches. The teeth are innervated by primary afferent fibres that have their peripheral endings in the pulp-dentine complex and also in the periodontal ligament. The fibres responsible for the conduction of pain (nociceptive fibres) are the Aδ and C fibres (Table 20.1). If endodontic intervention is required, it is important that these fibres are inhibited to facilitate effective treatment. Local anaesthetics are therefore necessary to reversibly block the sodium channels present in the nerve axon membrane. This prevents their depolarisation and transmission of a painful response to the cerebral cortex. A variety of dental local anaesthetics are available (Table 20.2).

Administration of local anaesthetic

To achieve enough duration and profound local anaesthesia:
- Apply topical anaesthetic gel
- More than one cartridge of anaesthetic may be required for irreversible pulpitis.
- Maxillary teeth can be anaethetised effectively with buccal and palatal infiltration (3 : 1 dosage).
- An inferior dental nerve block with Lidocaine is necessary to anaesthetise lower molars and second premolars. An additional buccal infiltration using Articaine is recommended to block the long buccal nerve.
- Avoiding the perception of pain in the first place is more effective than additional measures to increase the profoundness of the anaesthesia.
- Lower first premolars can be successfully anaesthetised with a mental nerve block.
- The mental nerve block will not always adequately anaesthetise lower incisors because of some crossover innervation from the contralateral incisive branch. These teeth can require a supplemental buccal and lingual infiltration.

Assessment of success of local anaesthetic

- The onset of modern local anaesthetics is rapid in normal conditions. In cases of irreversible pulpitis, longer waiting times and supplemental anaesthesia is required.
- Adequate anaesthesia is commonly assessed by asking patients if they can feel their lip, or assessing mucosal responsiveness with a sharp probe. However, the responses can be subjective and imprecise.
- An electric pulp tester or Endofrost can be used to test an adjacent vital asymptomatic tooth, with a negative response confirming the anaesthesia level. However, in cases of irreversible pulpitis, a negative response to the pulp tester is still no guarantee of full anaesthesia and the patient should be advised that further supplemental injections may be required.

Failure of local anaesthetic and alternative techniques

Dental anaesthesia can fail if there is insufficient volume, incorrect placement of the anaesthetic solution or if the dentist has not allowed adequate time for it to exert its effect. There may be accessory nerves requiring additional anaesthesia. In severe pulpal inflammation such as irreversible pulpitis, it is often more difficult to obtain anaesthesia. Reasons for this include the following:
- Inflamed tissue is acidic which reduces the amount of anaesthetic able to cross the nerve membrane.
- Inflamed pulp tissue has increased tetrodotoxin-resistant (TTX-R) sodium channels. Some anaesthetics are unable to block these effectively, therefore the nerves will still depolarise in response to noxious stimuli.
- Inflamed tissue has a lower threshold for excitation and is therefore more likely to depolarise in response to a noxious stimulus.
- Patients who are in pain are often more nervous. This can lower the pain threshold.

Lower molars are the most difficult to achieve adequate pulpal anaesthesia and if these teeth do not respond to an inferior alveolar nerve block and long buccal infiltration, a second nerve block can be tried in a slightly higher position using mepivacaine (which is able to block the TTX-R sodium channels). Anaesthetic can also be administered via intraosseous, intraligamentary or intrapulpal approaches.

Additional anaesthetic requirements for endodontic surgery

- Greater volumes of anaesthetic are required when performing surgery as anaesthesia is required over a larger area.
- Raising of a flap during surgery will also decrease the effectiveness of the anaesthetic because of its dilution by bleeding and irrigation of the area.
- Adrenaline-containing anaesthetics should be used if possible, and adequate time must be allowed for them to act, prior to commencing the surgical incisions. The adrenaline constricts the arterioles thereby reducing the blood flow to the surgical field to decrease perioperative bleeding. This improves visualisation during the procedure and prolongs the duration of the anaesthesia.

Adverse effects of local anaesthetic

- Adverse effects of local anaesthetic include cardiovascular effects as a result of adrenaline administration. The patient may experience tachycardia or a transient increase in blood pressure.
- Systemic effects such as muscle twitching, tremors and convulsions followed by sedation, hypotension and respiratory arrest can occur in local anaesthetic overdose.
- Long-term paraesthesia of the lingual or inferior alveolar nerve is a very rare complication of an inferior dental nerve block.
- Diploplia, ophthalmoplegia and amaurosis are very rare occurrences following inferior and posterior superior alveolar nerve blocks.

21 Pain management in endodontics

Figure 21.1 Ways that a hypochlorite accident can be reduced.

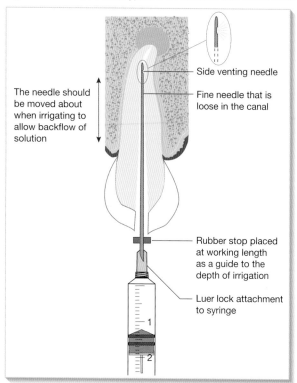

The needle should be moved about when irrigating to allow backflow of solution

Side venting needle

Fine needle that is loose in the canal

Rubber stop placed at working length as a guide to the depth of irrigation

Luer lock attachment to syringe

Box 21.1 Signs and symptoms of systemic infection.

Signs	Symptoms
• Raised temperature	• Malaise
• Hot flushed skin	• Nausea
• Increased heart rate	• Loss of appetite
• Low blood pressure	• Fatigue
• Swelling	

Figure 21.2 Predisposing factors for a postoperative flare up.

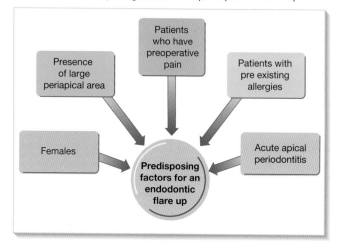

- Presence of large periapical area
- Patients who have preoperative pain
- Patients with pre existing allergies
- Females
- Acute apical periodontitis

Predisposing factors for an endodontic flare up

Figure 21.3 Causes of a postoperative flare up.

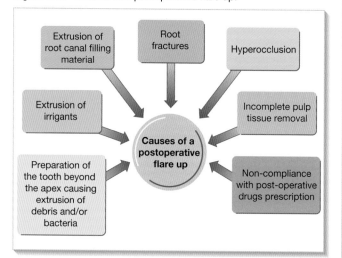

- Extrusion of root canal filling material
- Root fractures
- Hyperocclusion
- Extrusion of irrigants
- Incomplete pulp tissue removal
- Preparation of the tooth beyond the apex causing extrusion of debris and/or bacteria
- Non-compliance with post-operative drugs prescription

Causes of a postoperative flare up

Table 21.1 Advantages and disadvantages of the commonly prescribed antibiotics in endodontics.

Antibiotic	Advantages	Disadvantages
Amoxcyillin	• High antimicrobial activity for gram positive bacteria • Broad spectrum • Minimal side effects • Safe during pregnancy	• Some strains of bacteria have developed resistance to penicillins • Penicillin may be associated with type 1 hypersensitivity reactions (anaphalaxis)
Metronidazole	• Effective against obligate anaerobes • Resistance to metronidazole is uncommon	• Does not have as broad a spectrum of antimicrobial action as amoxicillin • Can be associated with unpleasant side effects including nausea and vomiting (especially after alcohol consumption) • Reacts with lithium-containing medications • Not advised in pregnant patients
Erythromycin	• Broad spectrum activity against facultative and anaerobic bacteria • Resistance is less common than for amoxicillin • Safe during pregnancy	• Gram negative bacteria are resistant to erythromycin • Common side effects include abdominal discomfort, diarrhoea, nausea and vomiting

Endodontology at a Glance. First Edition. Alix Davies, Federico Foschi and Shanon Patel. © 2019 John Wiley & Sons, Ltd. Published 2019 by John Wiley & Sons, Ltd.
Companion website: www.wiley.com/go/davies/endodontology

Pain from the oral structures is either odontogenic or non-odontogenic in origin (see Chapter 19). Emergency endodontic treatment may be required to manage patients who present with pain as a result of an acute pulpitis, acute apical periodontitis or an acute apical abscess. Pain can also occur during or after endodontic treatment. It is important that this is prevented where possible and, if it does occur, appropriate management ensues.

Management of acute pulpitis and acute apical periodontitis

Acute pulpitis and acute apical periodontitis is due to inflammation of the pulp and/or periapical tissues as a result of bacterial irritation (see Chapters 1 and 2).

- Patients presenting with pain require removal of this irritant.
- Management involves caries removal, followed by pulp extirpation and root canal debridement.
- A provisional dressing and filling should be placed to prevent reinfection.
- If full debridement is not possible because of inadequate time being available, or in cases where the patient presents with a 'hot pulp' that cannot be instrumented, the canal should be dressed with Odontopaste (steroid/antibiotic paste) to suppress pulpal inflammation.

Pain management for an acute apical abscess

When a patient attends with an acute apical abscess, management aims to establish surgical drainage and to remove the cause of the infection by root canal debridement.

- Antibiotics are only prescribed if there is evidence of spreading infection or systemic involvement (Box 21.1).
- Antibiotics must not be used as an alternative to dental intervention.
- Antibiotics may be required so supplement operative treatment in patients who are medically compromised because of systemic disease (e.g. HIV, leukaemia or poorly controlled diabetes).
- Patients should be assessed on an individual basis and antibiotics prescribed only where necessary. Antibiotics may be indicated when it is not possible to establish drainage or remove the cause of infection at an emergency appointment for patients in whom the infection is related to a root treated tooth.
- Antibiotics can be indicated in these patients to limit the local spread of infection, treat any systemic infection and bring about temporary symptomatic relief. In all cases, definitive treatment is required as soon as possible.
- Intraoral abscesses can be surgically drained to release pus and reduce the bacterial load. Using Endofrost on the abscess can reduce tenderness during incision with a scalpel.

Perioperative pain management

It is important to manage pain before and during endodontic treatment to maintain patient comfort and enable the operator to work effectively.

- The pain of the local anaesthetic injection should be eased by placement of topical anaesthetic, followed by the slow administration of prewarmed local anaesthetic solution to avoid excessive tissue distension. Palatal injections are more painful because of the low tissue compliance. Using the back of a mirror handle to press firmly on the area of the greater palatine foramen helps reduce tenderness. The upper anterior sextant is densely innervated, which can increase the pain experienced on injection. Massage of these tissues during the injection can reduce their sensitivity.
- Adequate time must be allowed for the anaesthetic to take effect before treatment is started (see Chapter 20). A bite block should also be offered to the patient to minimise jaw fatigue and aching during the lengthy procedure.
- A hypochlorite accident will cause perioperative and postoperative pain. This occurs if hypochlorite is extruded into the periradicular tissues via a perforation, or if hypochlorite is forced out of the apical foramen under pressure. Methods of reducing the risk of a hypochlorite accident are shown in Figure 21.1. If a hypochlorite accident occurs, treatment should be halted and additional local anaesthetic administered to the area. A cold compress should be applied alongside advice on pain relief, ideally with a combination of NSAIDs and paracetamol. Antibiotics can be given and the patient should be reviewed 24 hours later.

Postoperative pain management

Endodontic flare ups are acute episodes of pain and swelling that occur after a non-surgical root canal treatment. Certain preoperative factors (Figure 21.2) and treatment factors (Figure 21.3) can also make patients more susceptible to postoperative pain.

- An acute flare up can be minimised by confining the chemomechanical preparation to the root canal.
- Using a small file if carrying out patency filing.
- The pulp should be removed and the canals should be completely cleaned and shaped during the first appointment to reduce the bacteria remaining in the root canal.
- Careful technique and adoption of A crown down approach will minimise the bacterial load in any extruded debris.
- Occlusal reduction of the root treated tooth can also reduce postoperative discomfort.
- NSAIDs such as ibuprofen and where necessary supplemented with paracetamol is advised for the management of post-treatment pain subject to the no medical contraindications.
- Long acting local anaesthetics may be used to delay and/or reduce postoperative pain.
- Indiscriminate prescribing of post-treatment antibiotics is not routinely justified as flare ups occur in less than 10% of cases.
- If a patient develops a post-treatment flare up, he/she should be advised on pain relief, ensuring that the recommended dose limits are not exceeded.
- If there is swelling, reopening the tooth to establish drainage, and further instrumentation and irrigation can be required.
- Antibiotics should only be considered in immunocompromised patients or those with persistent or spreading infection.

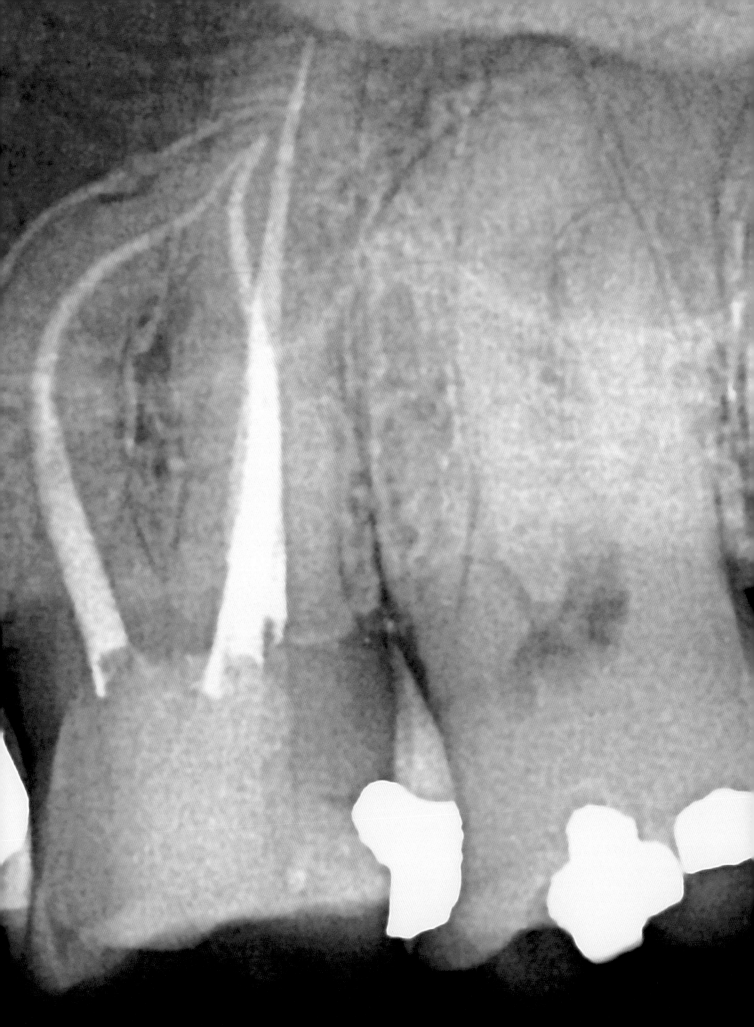

Outcome of endodontic treatment

Chapters

22 Outcome of root canal treatment

Figure 22.1 Reducing coronal tooth tissue with loss of the marginal ridges leads to greater risk of tooth fracture and decreased survival.

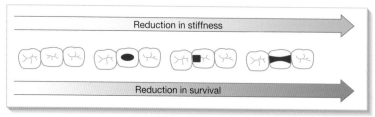

Figure 22.2 The position of the tooth in the arch and the number of proximal contacts influences the survival of the root treated tooth.

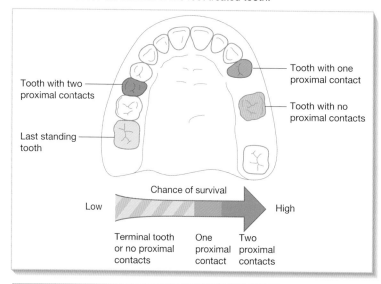

Box 22.1 Factors affecting success rates.

Preoperative factors that reduce the prognosis of root canal treatment
- Medical history – diabetics or immunosuppressed patients
- Presence of a periapical area
- Presence of a fistula
- Pre-operative radiolucency
- Multirooted teeth
- Limited amount of residual tooth structure
- Lack of a ferrule
- Terminal position of tooth in the arch
- Cracked tooth
- Previously ledged or blocked root canals that cannot be bypassed
- Previous perforations
- Previous well-performed root canal treatments that have still failed

Perioperative factors that improve the prognosis of root canal treatment
- Experienced clinician
- Use of magnification
- Appropriate choice of irrigating solutions
- Instrumentation of all canals to length
- Obturation of all canals to within 2 mm of the apex
- Prevention of procedural errors such as ledges and blocked canals

Postoperative factors that reduce the prognosis of the root canal treatment
- Defective coronal seal
- Missing cuspal coverage restoration
- Use of the tooth as an abutment
- Uncontrolled periodontal disease
- Recurrent caries
- Parafunctional activity

Endodontology at a Glance. First Edition. Alix Davies, Federico Foschi and Shanon Patel. © 2019 John Wiley & Sons, Ltd. Published 2019 by John Wiley & Sons, Ltd.
Companion website: www.wiley.com/go/davies/endodontology

A successful outcome is when there is an absence of pain, swelling and other symptoms, there is no sinus tract, no loss of function and there is radiological evidence of a normal periodontal ligament space around the root. Outcome can also be measured by assessing the survival time of the tooth in the mouth after treatment. Whilst this is could be considered a more crude assessment, it is often more relevant to the patient. Outcomes have been determined by studies that follow up patients over a period of time to determine their success or survival.

Success rates of root canal treatment vary from 60% to 100% for primary root canal treatments when cases were assessed with periapical radiography. However, when the outcome is assessed using cone beam computed tomography (CBCT), a lower initial rate of healing is demonstrated. Retreatment cases show lower success rates than initial treatments.

The factors that influence the outcome can be divided into preoperative, perioperative and postoperative factors (Box 22.1).

Preoperative factors

- The presence of a periapical radiolucency is considered to be one of the most important factors affecting the outcome as this indicates that there is a signifcant level of bacteria within the root canal system.
- The presence of a sinus tract is often associated with an increased complexity of bacterial species which is harder to eliminate.
- Lesions with periodontal involvement have lower success rates as a good outcome relies not only on chemomechanical instrumentation of the root canals, but also on adequate root surface debridement and patient cooperation.
- Multirooted teeth tend to have a poorer success rate than single rooted teeth. This is because of the more complex morphology of multirooted teeth.
- The risk of a tooth fracturing and needing extraction increases when there is minimal coronal tooth tissue (Figure 22.1) or in teeth with pre-existing cracks which are more likely to propagate.
- The risk of fracture increases if the tooth is the most distal tooth remaining in an arch, or it does not have two proximal contacts with adjacent teeth (Figure 22.2).
- Retreatment of teeth where the canals have previously been ledged or blocked, or there are other procedural errors such as perforations can prevent the operator accessing and disinfecting the apical portion of the canal. The prognosis is thus reduced.
- Conversely, patients in whom treatment was initially performed to a high clinical standard but has still failed have a lower chance of being successful on a second attempt because of the likely presence of virulent bacteria or difficult apical root canal anatomy.

Perioperative factors

- The greater the experience of the operator, the higher the chance of success, especially when dealing with complex cases.
- Magnification is often used by these operators and can aid localisation of additional canals such as the MB2 to increase the likelihood of a favourable outcome.
- Sodium hypochlorite is the most effective irrigant as it possesses broad spectrum antimicrobial activity and is able to dissolve organic material such as the necrotic pulp (see Chapter 12).
- Calcium hydroxide can be used as a root canal medicament to decrease the remaining bacterial load after chemomechanical preparation with sodium hypochlorite. It is especially useful in patients with internal resorption or where there is continued exudate from the canals (see Chapter 13). However, there is no difference in the outcome between cases completed in one visit, and those completed in multiple visits with an interappointment dressing.
- One of the main perioperative factors affecting the outcome of root canal treatment is the use of rubber dam as it facilitates the use of sodium hypochlorite.
- In teeth with a periapical radiolucency, instrumentation to the working length and ensuring patency are paramount to success.
- Any procedural error that prevents full chemomechanical debridement will reduce the success rate of the treatment.
- Favourable outcomes of root canal treated teeth in patients with a preoperative periapical area have been shown to be highest when the canal is filled to within 2 mm of the apex.
- Under and overfilled canals have shown reduced success rates.

Postoperative factors

- It is important that the root canal system is sealed coronally to prevent bacterial recontamination.
- Tooth fracture after treatment is the main cause of extraction of root filled teeth. Posterior teeth that have lost one or both marginal ridges, and/or present with microcracks, should be restored with a cuspal coverage restoration.
- Teeth subject to increased forces are more likely to fail. These include those used as abutments for bridges or dentures, and also teeth in patients with parafunction.
- Recurrent caries and uncontrolled periodontal disease also reduce the survival of root treated teeth.

23 Outcome of root canal surgery

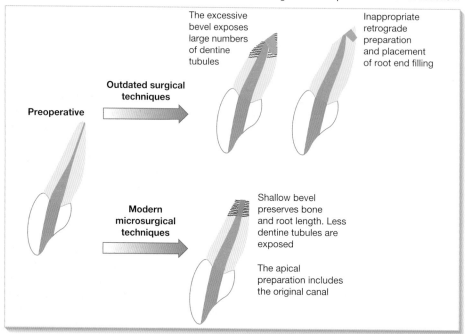

Figure 23.1 Comparison of traditional and current microsurgical techniques for root end resection.

Preoperative

Outdated surgical techniques

The excessive bevel exposes large numbers of dentine tubules

Inappropriate retrograde preparation and placement of root end filling

Modern microsurgical techniques

Shallow bevel preserves bone and root length. Less dentine tubules are exposed

The apical preparation includes the original canal

Box 23.1 Factors that affect the outcome of root canal surgery.

Preoperative factors that affect the prognosis of root end surgery
- Medical history
- Case selection
- Tooth type
- Initial surgery or repeat surgery
- Size of the periapical lesion
- Amount of tooth tissue remaining

Perioperative factors that affect the prognosis of root end surgery
- Operator experience
- Use of the microscope
- Flap design
- Amount of bone removal
- Root end preparation technique
- Root end obturation material

Postoperative factors that affect the prognosis of root end surgery
- Cuspal coverage restorations
- Use of the tooth as an abutment
- Periodontal disease
- Recurrent caries
- Parafunctional activity

Endodontology at a Glance. First Edition. Alix Davies, Federico Foschi and Shanon Patel. © 2019 John Wiley & Sons, Ltd. Published 2019 by John Wiley & Sons, Ltd.
Companion website: www.wiley.com/go/davies/endodontology

A successful outcome for root end surgery occurs when there is an absence of pain, swelling and other symptoms, there is no sinus tract, no loss of function and there is radiological evidence of a normal periodontal ligament space around the root.

Outcomes have been determined by studies that follow up patients over a period of time. Most of the studies assessing root end surgery have been performed by specialists in oral surgery or endodontics. Current root end microsurgery techniques performed on appropriate patients have a success rate of up to 90%.

The factors that influence the outcome of root end surgery can be divided into preoperative, perioperative and postoperative factors (Box 23.1).

Preoperative factors

• Apical root surgery had a poor outcome in the past. However, this was because case selection was poor and it was used in substitution for the provision of a good orthograde root filling. In most cases, teeth with poorly fitting coronal restorations and inadequate root canal fillings should initially undergo retreatment to ensure that the canal is fully disinfected prior to placement of a good root filling and coronal restoration.

• Anterior teeth have a higher success rate than posterior teeth because of better access for the surgical procedure.

• A tooth undergoing its first surgical procedure has a better prognosis than one that is to undergo retreatment. The reasons for this are likely to be a result of previous poor surgical technique which involved bevelling the root end or perforation of the root leaving the operator little remaining root to prepare and fill at the second surgical attempt.

• A tooth with a large periapical lesion will have had more bone loss and will therefore take longer to heal than one with a smaller lesion.

• As with conventional root canal treatment, it is pointless performing root end surgery on a tooth that is unrestorable. It is important that the tooth has a good coronal seal and a cuspal coverage restoration if necessary.

Perioperative factors

• Use of the dental operating microscope has revolutionised the way in which surgery is performed and has increased the probability of success. It has allowed for a reduction in the size of the osteotomy, resulting in shorter healing times.

• Prior to microsurgical techniques, root-end preparation included a bevel to improve access for placement of the root end filling. However, this bevel exposes more dentine tubules to the surrounding tissues. Root end surgery now aims to keep the root end as flat as possible to reduce the exposure of dentine tubules and therefore egress of bacterial contents. These shallower resection angles also conserve more cortical bone and preserve root length.

• Using microsurgical ultrasonic instruments to penetrate and shape the apical root canal allows a more conservative preparation which is easier to fill. They reduce the incidence of perforations and cracks which were caused by larger burs. In addition, root end preparation using traditional techniques often did not actually incorporate the canal being prepared (Figure 23.1). This contrasts with microsurgical techniques where there is improved visualisation, making it is far easier to prepare the root end within the confines of the canal whilst also including any isthmuses and lateral canals.

• Amalgam has been replaced by IRM or MTA, both of which demonstrate superior success rates (see Chapter 18). Other materials such as composites have been used as root filling materials in the past but are no longer advised because of the difficulty in obtaining a dry root surface for bonding. Glass ionomer-based filling materials are also no longer recommended because of their water absorption and breakdown in the moist environment.

• Whilst carrying out root end surgery, it is important to design the flap to ensure there is adequate access. The flap should be protected during the procedure and should maintain hydration. Retractors should rest on the bone and not the flap to reduce the risk of tearing or crushing it as this will delay healing.

Postoperative factors

• Teeth that have had root end surgery have the same cuspal coverage requirements as those that have had conventional root canal treatment.

• As there is less root remaining after surgery and less bone support, the use of these teeth as abutments for fixed or removable prostheses significantly lowers their long-term prognosis.

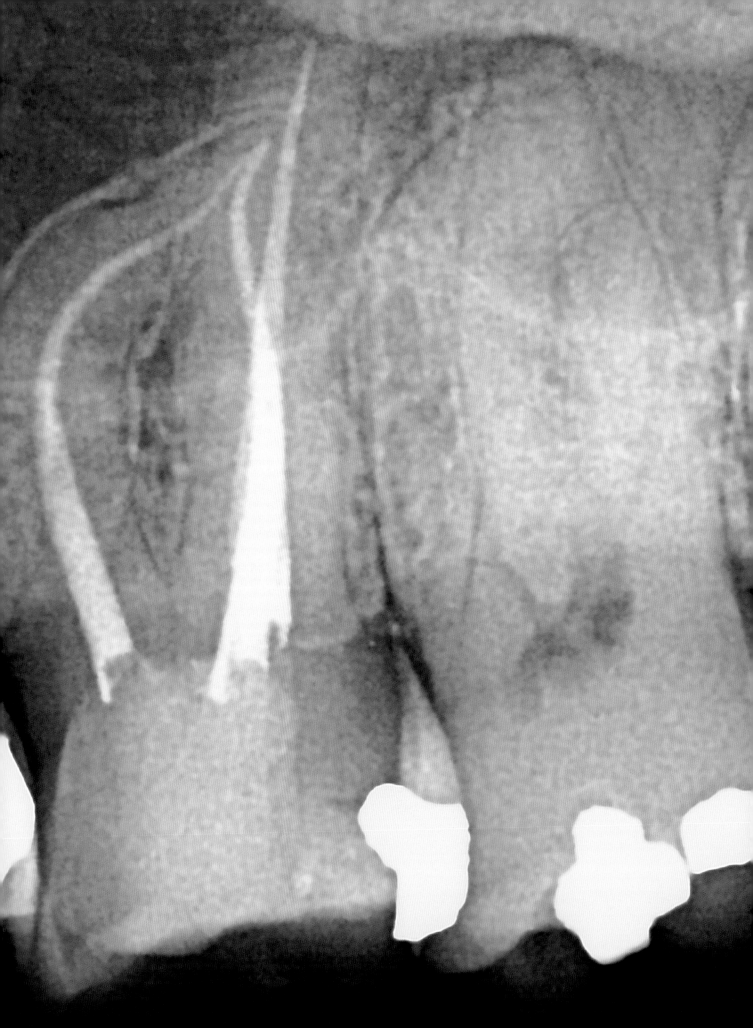

Endodontology and other aspects of dentistry

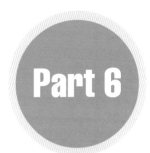

Part 6

Chapters

24 Endodontic–periodontic interface

Table 24.1 Features of lesions of endodontic and periodontal origin.

	Primary endodontic disease	Primary endodontic disease with secondary periodontal involvement	Primary periodontal disease	Primary periodontal disease with secondary endodontic involvement	Concomitant and true combined endodontic and periodontal disease
Diagram	(a)	(b)	(c)	(d)	(e)
	⟶ Pathway of inflammation ◯◯ Plaque/calculus deposits ▬ Lateral/furcal canals				
Response to vitality testing	Negative	Negative	Positive	Negative	Negative
Restorative status	Deep caries or restorations present or a history of trauma	Deep caries or restorations present or a history of trauma	Not relevant to the disease – the teeth may be minimally restored	Not relevant to the disease – the teeth may be minimally restored	Deep caries or restorations present or a history of trauma
Periodontal pocketing	Deep localised pocket only if pus is draining via the periodontal ligament. There may be no pocket	Localised pocket which is wider and associated with plaque and calculus	Multiple pockets that are wide	Multiple pockets that are wide	Multiple pockets that are wide
Periapical radiograph findings	There may be a periapical area but there will be no marginal bone loss	Presence of a periapical area and localised marginal bone loss causing a vertical bony defect	Generalised bone loss. No periapical area will be present	Generalised bone loss which will be extensive and deep around the tooth in question. There may also be a periapical area	Generalised bone loss which will be extensive and deep around the tooth in question. There will also be a periapical area
Treatment	Root canal treatment only	Root canal treatment followed by periodontal therapy	Periodontal therapy only	Root canal treatment followed by periodontal therapy	Root canal treatment followed by periodontal therapy

Endodontology at a Glance. First Edition. Alix Davies, Federico Foschi and Shanon Patel. © 2019 John Wiley & Sons, Ltd. Published 2019 by John Wiley & Sons, Ltd.
Companion website: www.wiley.com/go/davies/endodontology

Most cases of endodontic and periodontal disease occur in isolation. However, there are times when the presence of one can facilitate development of the other. In these situations, the disease is classified according to its primary cause (Table 24.1). However, diagnosis is often challenging because both diseases may present in similar ways. It is therefore essential that a good history, clinical and radiographic examinations are performed. The prognosis is reduced for teeth with both pulpal and periodontal problems as it relies on the success of both endodontic and periodontal procedures. Whilst endodontic treatment relies purely on the operator to ensure adequate chemomechanical debridement and obturation of the canals, periodontal treatment requires meticulous debridement by the operator, but also patient cooperation and compliance. Long-term periodontal maintenance is also necessary in patients with periodontally involved teeth.

Primary endodontic disease

Primary endodontic disease is caused by inflammatory changes to the pulp, most commonly caused by trauma or caries. If it remains untreated, bacteria will spread to the apical portions and cause inflammation and result in loss of the surrounding periapical bone. Pus can accumulate and drain via the path of least resistance which can be the periodontal ligament space. Although a probe or gutta percha point can be inserted through the sinus to the apex of the tooth, there is initially no increased probing depth around the rest of the tooth. However, if plaque and calculus build up around the sinus opening, they will cause gingival inflammation which can progress to the marginal bone and periodontal ligament, leading to periodontal breakdown. This is classified as a primary endodontic disease with secondary periodontal involvement. A furcal or lateral canal in a tooth with an infected necrotic pulp, or a perforation that is not immediately repaired, can also result in secondary periodontal disease. Hairline cracks and vertical root fractures can simulate the single spot pocketing of a draining intrasulcular sinus.

The tooth will respond negatively to vitality testing for primary endodontic lesions. The teeth are likely to be extensively restored, carious and/or demonstrate cracks. Those with additional secondary periodontal involvement can show accumulation of plaque and calculus and the periapical radiographs may show angular bony defects around the tooth involved. Bone levels are often normal around the other teeth.

Primary endodontic lesions should initially be managed by root canal treatment. If the lesion has secondary periodontal involvement, periodontal therapy is also necessary.

Primary periodontal disease

Primary periodontal disease is caused by marginal periodontal inflammation as a result of accumulation of plaque and calculus in susceptible individuals. As the periodontal atttachment progresses apically, lateral and apical canals are exposed to bacteria residing in the gingival sulcus. Bacteria are also thought to enter via the dentine tubules. However, this would be uncommon in a tooth with a healthy pulp because of the pulpal hydrostatic pressure producing an outward fluid movement in the dentine tubules which would limit bacterial ingress. The bacteria can stimulate pulpal inflammation and necrosis. This is classified as primary periodontic disease with secondary endodontic involvement. Periodontal scaling and root planning also cause pulpal inflammation by removing cementum to expose the dentine tubules as well as disrupting the blood supply entering the pulp via a lateral or accessory foramina. However, the occurrence of pulpal problems in this manner is very rare.

In primary periodontal lesions, the tooth is likely to be associated with plaque and calculus and have generalised deep probing depths. Generalised horizontal marginal bone loss can be identified on the periapical radiographs. The tooth may be minimally restored and should respond positively to vitality testing. However, if there is secondary endodontic involvement, the tooth provides a negative response to vitality testing and there will be periapical bone loss in addition to the marginal bone loss.

Primary periodontal lesions require periodontal therapy. If there is secondary endodontic involvement, root canal treatment is required and this should be performed first.

Concomitant and true combined disease

Occasionally, a tooth with endodontic disease is also independently periodontally involved. This is known as concomitant pulpal and periodontal disease if there is no clinical evidence that one disease has caused the other and clinical and radiographic examination show the periodontic and endodontic lesions to be separate entities. Once both intrabony lesions coalesce, the disease can be classified as true combined endodontic and periodontic disease.

In these patients, the clinical examination shows a nonvital tooth with a likely build up of plaque and calculus as well as generalised probing depths. A periapical shows horizontal bone loss with an angular defect around the tooth affected with endodontic disease. There will be periapical bone loss. In these patients, both endodontic and periodontal therapy are required for healing to occur.

Management of persistent disease

If disease still persists after meticulous endodontic and periodontal therapy, alternative treatment approaches should be considered:

1 Root resections or hemisections may be indicated in multi-rooted teeth where one or more roots are considered unsavable. Teeth should be assessed carefully to confirm that the root is accessible for resection and is not fused.

The restorability and occlusal loading on the tooth must also be checked to ensure that the tooth will still function with reduced radicular support. Ideally, a tooth that is to undergo root resection should undergo root canal treatment first, followed by resection, sealing of the root stump with a calcium silicate material, and recontouring of the root to prevent creation of a food and plaque trap that would be inaccessible to cleaning.

2 Extraction and, if necessary, replacement with an implant, bridge or denture.

25 Endodontic–orthodontic interface

Table 25.1 Factors that predict greater resorption during orthodontic treatment of a vital tooth.

Root morphology	Blunt or pipette shaped roots
Habits	• Nail biting • Digit sucking
Iatrogenic factors	• Prolonged treatment • Excessive orthodontic forces • Extrusive orthodontic movements • Intrusive orthodontic movements • Increased amount of tooth movement required • Torquing movements with rectangular arch wires • Intermaxillary elastic traction

Box 25.1 Factors that predict greater resorption in a tooth that has been previously traumatised.

- **Severity of trauma** Intrusive luxations and avulsions present the greatest risk of resorption
- **Diameter of apical foramen** The larger the apical diameter, the lower the risk of resorption
- **Presence or history of resorption** Teeth with signs of resorption before orthodontic treatment may be at increased risk of resorption during orthodontic treatment.

Endodontology at a Glance. First Edition. Alix Davies, Federico Foschi and Shanon Patel. © 2019 John Wiley & Sons, Ltd. Published 2019 by John Wiley & Sons, Ltd.
Companion website: www.wiley.com/go/davies/endodontology

Orthodontic treatment may influence the pulpal and peri-apical status of a tooth, especially if the pulp has had previous insults such as a deep filling or trauma. A combined orthodontic and endodontic approach may be required to plan complex restorative cases as well as determine the management of traumatised teeth. The indications of orthodontics to manage luxated teeth is described in Chapter 34. It is therefore important for both specialities to have an understanding of the other and recognise situations when a joint approach is required.

Effect of orthodontic treatment on the pulp and periapical tissues

Orthodontic movement of teeth can cause minor pulpal inflammatory changes. This usually has no consequence. However, the inflammatory changes can have a more profound effect in pulps that are already compromised (i.e. inflamed) as a result of previous caries or trauma. Devitalisation of healthy pulps is unusual during the course of orthodontic treatment. However, if excessive force is used, the blood supply to the tooth can be compromised which can lead to pulpal necrosis.

Orthodontic movement relies on the coupling of osteoblastic and osteoclastic cells to remodel bone. Some mediators produced during bone remodelling are the same as those released by inflammatory cells which stimulate bone resorption in apical periodontitis. In teeth with pre-existing apical periodontitis, orthodontic movement can increase the levels of these mediators, causing more bone loss at the apex of the tooth and more unpredictable movement. It is therefore important that, prior to commencing orthodontic treatment, the pulpal and periapical status of all teeth are assessed to ensure that both vital and root treated teeth do not display signs of chronic apical periodontitis. In the absence of apical periodontitis, there are no contraindications to orthodontic tooth movement of root filled teeth. Teeth that display chronic apical periodontitis should be treated or retreated prior to orthodontic movement. The orthodontic treatment can then be started once any postoperative discomfort has subsided.

Historically, calcium hydroxide was placed in the root canal for the duration of orthodontic treatment. However, long-term use of calcium hydroxide has been shown to weaken the tooth. Immediate obturation is preferable (see Chapter 27).

Effect of orthodontic treatment on the diagnosis and process of root canal treatment

- Diagnosis can be challenging in patients who are having orthodontic treatment as it can be confounded by the discomfort of the tooth movement.

- Isolation of the tooth with rubber dam is difficult when arch wires are in situ and it may be easier to request temporary removal of these.
- If wires are kept in situ, use of damming material (e.g. Oraseal) is recommended to improve isolation.
- If the tooth is at an angle, it is important that this is identified so that the access cavity is cut appropriately and perforation is avoided.
- Extensive apical root resorption can affect the apex locator readings.

Effect of orthodontic treatment on root resorption

Small amounts of resorption occur in most patients undergoing fixed appliance orthodontic treatment. Occasionally more extensive resorption occurs; this is more common in upper incisors. Factors that increase the risk of root resorption in a healthy tooth are described in Table 25.1. Orthodontic treatment is a claimed cause of external cervical root resorption, however, there is no strong evidence for this.

Effect of orthodontic treatment on traumatised teeth

A traumatized tooth can usually be moved orthodontically with minimal risk of resorption, provided the pulp has not been severely compromised (inflamed or infected). If there is evidence of pulpal demise, appropriate endodontic management is necessary prior to orthodontic treatment. Factors predicting a greater than normal amount of root resorption in the orthodontic movement of previously traumatized teeth are shown in Box 25.1.

If a tooth has undergone a traumatic episode, any active orthodontic treatment should be stopped and baseline radiographs should be taken. If any endodontic treatment is required then this should be carried out.

A further periapical should be taken 3 months later and then, provided that there are no periapical changes and the tooth responds normally to clinical tests, tooth movement can be continued.

Teeth with healed fractures can be moved orthodontically if the tooth is clinically and radiographically healthy.

Role of orthodontics in endodontic and restorative treatment planning

Where there is any doubt on the long-term prognosis of a tooth, an orthodontic opinion may be required to consider extraction of the tooth and space closure. This is common for first molars in children where the space can be closed by mesial movement of the second and third molars.

26 Restoration of the endodontically treated tooth

Figure 26.1 Graph showing the approximate survival rates of root filled teeth that have been restored with and without cuspal coverage restorations.

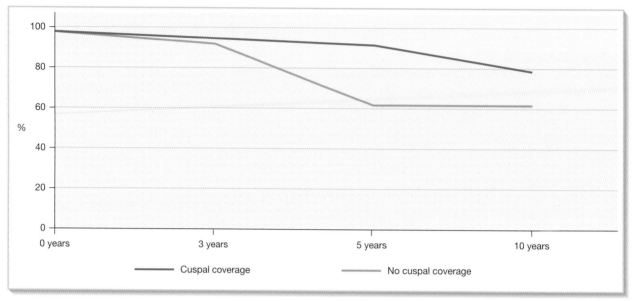

Table 26.1 Advantages and disadvantages of prefabricated and laboratory made posts.

	Prefabricated posts	Laboratory made posts
Advantages	• Less preparation of the canal is required, preserving tooth structure • Glass fibre posts can bond to the root surface to create a good seal • Posts can be placed immediately after the root treatment, therefore maintaining the coronal seal • Glass fibre posts are tooth coloured, resulting in improved aesthetics • Only one chairside visit is required and there are no laboratory fees, making this a cheaper option	• Root canals are not perfect circles so the post can be constucted to fit the canal • If there is very little ferrule, the cast post can provide extra rigidity • The angle of the crown relative to the root can be easily adjusted. This is harder to do with direct posts • Removal is relatively easy using ultrasonics to disrupt the lute
Disadvantages	• Removal of fibre posts can be difficult	• Requires more chairside and laboratory time • More tooth tissue must be removed to create a path of insertion. This can result in the loss of any ferrule present and increase the risk of fracture • Placement of a temporary post crown is required whilst the laboratory constructs the definitive restoration. • Temporary posts have a poor seal • Failure is often associated with fracture of the tooth and extraction of the tooth is inevitable • The metal can cause shine through and be harder to mask with porcelain restorations

Box 26.1 Ideal characteristics of the core material.

• Dimensional stability
• High compressive and flexural strength
• Easy to manipulate and adapt straight away to cut a crown preparation
• Short setting time
• Setting is not affected by root canal sealers such as zinc oxide eugenol
• Material should be a slightly different shade to the dentine to allow its removal if necessary

Endodontology at a Glance. First Edition. Alix Davies, Federico Foschi and Shanon Patel. © 2019 John Wiley & Sons, Ltd. Published 2019 by John Wiley & Sons, Ltd.
Companion website: www.wiley.com/go/davies/endodontology

Once root canal treatment has been completed, the tooth must be permanenty sealed coronally to prevent bacterial ingress and (re-)contamination of the root canal. It must then be restored to its functional and aesthetic form. In posterior teeth this usually involves the placement of a core of restorative material, followed by a cuspal coverage restoration (e.g. onlay or crown). Ideal characteristics of the core material are shown in Box 26.1.

Amalgam has a high compressive and tensile strength adequate for many core build ups. The main disadvantage is the slow set, which prevents the core immediately being prepared for a temporary crown. It is not adhesive and so will not reinforce the tooth and microleakage can occur. Amalgam is no longer advised as a core material as there are better alternatives.

Resin-modified glass ionomers have moderate strength and adhere to dentine. However, they show hygroscopic expansion and should therefore only be used as small to moderate size cores. Their set is not inhibited by eugenol containing cements, thus making them an ideal layer to place between the root filling and a composite core.

Composites are becoming increasingly popular as cores. They have good mechanical strength and can be bonded to tooth tissue and to many types of post. Composite is easy to manipulate and sets immediately, thus allowing tooth preparation for a crown if necessary. The composite should be placed incrementally to minimise shrinkage on polymerization. The recently introduced bulk fill composites are prone to excessive shrinkage. Eugenol-based sealers can inhibit setting of the composite and any residual sealer must be removed from the access cavity prior to composite placement.

Placement of posts

A post is required if the amount of tooth structure remaining is not sufficient to support or retain a core. Posts do not strengthen the residual tooth structure. Posts are either preformed (direct post systems) or must be constructed by a laboratory technician. The advantages and disadvantages of each are shown in Table 26.1. Glass fibre post systems have superseded direct metal posts with the advantage that they have a module of elasticity closer to dentine, and can be cemented into the root canal space predictably in one single appointment. Many post systems now are adapted to the common tapers of the canals and are easy to place. The most common cause of failure associated with fibre post systems is post decementation. Conversely, root fracture is the main mode of failure of the metal posts, rendering the tooth unsalvageable.

Cuspal coverage restorations

Root treated teeth are at increased risk of fracture compared with their counterparts that have an intact nerve supply:

- Teeth requiring root canal treatment often have large amounts of decay or/are extensively restored and therefore have little natural tooth remaining. Loss of the marginal ridges reduces the tooth's resistance to fracture (see Chapter 22).
- Irrigants and medicaments can alter the strength and elasticity of the dentine.
- Parafunctional habits, may lead to the formation of hairline cracks in unrestored posterior teeth that can propagate in the absence of cuspal protection.
- A root treated tooth has no proprioceptive feedback and therefore can be subjected to increased biting forces.

Cuspal coverage restorations are therefore recommended in premolars and molars that do not have intact marginal ridges. They significantly increase the survival of root treated teeth (Figure 26.1). The timing of the indirect restoration must be balanced between establishing that the treatment is likely to be successful, whilst ensuring the tooth does not fracture or develop microleakage in the interim period. Asymptomatic teeth with no clinical or radiographic signs of endodontic or periodontal disease that have been treated to a technically satisfactory standard should be permanently restored within 1-2 weeks. Orthodontic bands, temporary crowns or cuspal coverage composite restorations should be placed to minimise the risk of fracture of the tooth in the interim period. The patient should also be advised to avoid eating hard foods on the root treated tooth until the definitive restoration is in place.

Use of root treated teeth as abutments

Teeth used as abutments for bridges and dentures receive an increased loading in function. This stress is greater if the bridge is of a cantilever design, or if the tooth is the distal abutment for a partial denture. Therefore, wherever possible, root filled teeth should be avoided as abutments. If one is to be used, it is important that there is adequate remaining sound tooth tissue for a ferrule, the root is an appropriate size to support the additional load and that the tooth is restored with a cuspal coverage restoration.

Parafunction and eccentric occlusal loading can lead to an excessive load on root canal treated abutment, therefore a thorough occlusion analysis should be carried out during the treatment planning.

27 Paediatric endodontics

Figure 27.1 Properties of Bioceramic Cements.

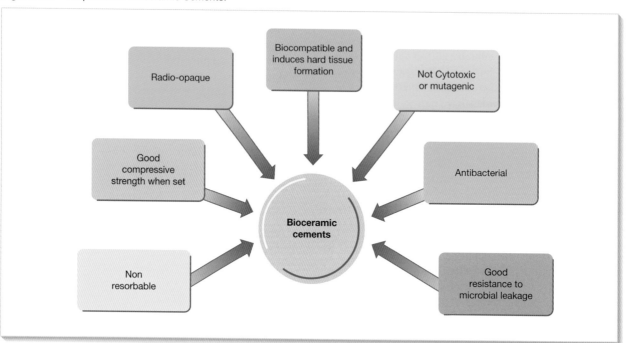

Figure 27.2 Radiographs showing the stages of root canal treatment in an upper incisor with an immature open apex. (a) Preoperative radiograph of UL1 showing a periapical lesion and immature open apex. (b) The canal is chemomechanically prepared and a working length radiograph is taken to confirm the canal length. (c) The canal is dried and MTA is placed with a plugger into the apical 2–4 mm of the canal. A radiograph is taken to confirm the correct apical positioning. (d) The canal is filled with 4–7 mm of MTA. (e) Gutta percha can be used to obturate the remaining canal or composite can be placed in the canal to bond to and reinforce the thin walls.

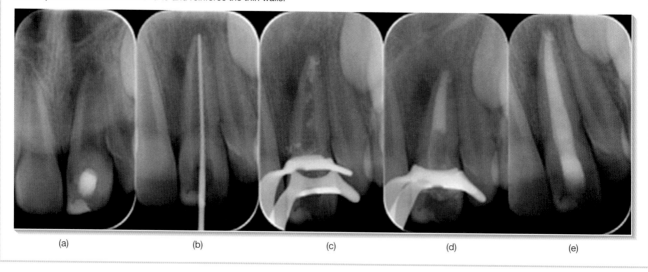

(a)   (b)   (c)   (d)   (e)

Endodontology at a Glance. First Edition. Alix Davies, Federico Foschi and Shanon Patel. © 2019 John Wiley & Sons, Ltd. Published 2019 by John Wiley & Sons, Ltd.
Companion website: www.wiley.com/go/davies/endodontology

Immature permanent teeth that are carious and/or have suffered trauma may require endodontic management. Correct diagnosis and treatment planning are essential to determine the best plan for the individual patient. This may involve an orthodontic opinion aiming to limit further trauma by reducing excessive overjets, or timed extractions of grossly carious first molars to allow mesial eruption of the second molars into this space (see Chapter 25).

Intensive diet advice and oral hygiene instruction are necessary for children who present with dental caries. Custom made mouthguards should be recommended to children involved in contact sports.

Diagnosis of endodontic problems

The diagnosis of endodontic problems in children can be challenging. Whilst some children present with an extensive pain history, others have no pain despite evidence of considerable decay.

The clinical examination may be harder to perform in apprehensive children, and pulp testing is unreliable in immature permanent teeth. False negative responses can occur in undamaged normal teeth because of incomplete formation of the root apex and maturation of the nerve supply. In these cases, cold testing with Endofrost can be more reliable than using an electric pulp tester. Conversely, a false positive response can be obtained in a young apprehensive patient when the pulp is actually necrotic.

Good quality periapicals are necessary although interpretation of periapical pathology is complicated by incompletely formed immature roots. It is advisable to compare the root formation of the tooth with a suspected endodontic problem with the contralateral tooth (providing this is considered healthy) to aid diagnosis and treatment planning. If there is any doubt regarding the endodontic status of the pulp, pulp preservation techniques should be used to maintain vitality rather than risk commencing root canal treatment unnecessarily.

Pulp preservation techniques

A root canal treated tooth is more susceptible to fracture than one with an intact nerve supply (see Chapter 26). An immature root treated tooth has a greater risk of fracture as the root may have very thin walls and a reduced crown to root ratio. Root canal treatment is often challenging because of large open apices that provide no resistance against compaction of the root filling.

Behavioural management of young patients during long treatment sessions can be demanding. It is therefore important that every effort is taken to preserve pulp vitality until dentine development is complete. Apexogenesis involves the use of techniques that aim to maintain healthy apical pulp tissue. This encourages physiological root development with dentine deposition strengthening the canal walls. Continued apical maturation will produce a closed apex. Techniques include indirect or direct pulp capping and pulpotomies (see Chapters 8 and 32).

Apexification

Apexification is the artificial closure of the apex of an immature non-vital tooth. It was previously achieved by placing calcium hydroxide in the canal. This dressing was refreshed every 3–6 months until a mineralised bridge was evident radiographically at the apex. This provided an apical stop to facilitate condensation of the root canal filling. However, it had the disadvantages of long treatment times (up to 18 months) and multiple visits. Frequent changes of calcium hydroxide dressings, and their placement over an extended time period, are also considered to biomechanically alter the dentine structure (i.e. deproteinisation of collagen) and increase the risk of root fracture.

The current gold standard in the treatment of incomplete apices of permanent teeth is to create an apical plug with a setting calcium silicate material. Bioceramic silicate materials like Biodentine and Mineral Trioxide Aggregate (MTA) set in the presence of moisture. They are sterile and biocompatible, inducing hard tissue formation on its surface. They are non-toxic and form a good seal with the root canal walls which resists marginal leakage (Figure 27.1); however, they are virtually impossible to remove (re-treat). Earlier produced grey MTA formulations caused some staining but newer white MTA formulations minimise this effect. A detailed informed consent should be gained to prewarn patients of possible discoloration and that internal bleaching might be required in the future.

Once the canal has been chemomechanically prepared, it should be dried. The presence of pus or blood draining from the periapical lesion into the canal can affect the setting of the material. An intermediate dressing with calcium hydroxide should be considered in these conditions.

Bioceramic cements should be mixed with distilled water and placed in small increments at the apex of the tooth using endodontic pluggers. Once a 4-mm increment is in place, a radiograph should be taken to confirm it has been placed in the correct position and is free of voids (Figure 27.2). Presence of voids into the plug can be addressed by ultrasonically activating a plugger in contact with the material. If apical surgery is envisioned, then a deeper filling (7-8mm) of MTA or Biodentine may be indicated to limit surgery to an apical root resection.

Restoration

Wherever possible, anterior teeth should be restored with direct composite resin. Indirect restorations such as veneers or full cuspal coverage crowns should be avoided to minimise the unnecessary removal of tooth structure unless there is an overarching cosmetic need. Posterior teeth that do not have intact marginal ridges require cuspal coverage restorations (see Chapter 26).

28 Endodontics in the older population

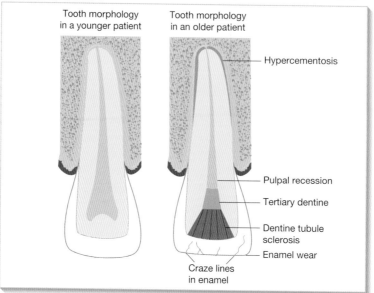

Figure 28.1 Changes in cement–dentinal junction position with increasing age.

Tooth morphology in a younger patient

Tooth morphology in an older patient

- Hypercementosis
- Pulpal recession
- Tertiary dentine
- Dentine tubule sclerosis
- Enamel wear
- Craze lines in enamel

Table 28.1 Commonly used drugs in endodontics and their possible interactions with other medicines.

	Drugs prescribed during endodontic treatment	Possible interacting drugs	Possible side effect	Management strategies
Local anaesthetic	Local anaesthetics containing adrenaline	Beta-blockers (e.g. atenolol, propanolol)	Hypertension	Limit the dosage or use adrenaline-free local anaesthetic
		Tricyclic antidepressants (e.g. imipramine, amitriptyline)	Increased adrenergic response	Limit the dosage or use adrenaline-free local anaesthetic
Pain relief	NSAIDs (e.g. ibuprofen)	Anticoagulants (warfarin, coumarins)	Increased risk of bleeding	Short-term use of NSAIDs or consult their GP
		ACE inhibitors (e.g. ramipril, captopril)	Hypertension	Short-term use of NSAIDs or consult their GP
		Aspirin	Increased risk of bleeding	Avoid use of NSAIDs
		Beta-blockers (e.g. atenolol, propanolol)	Hypertension	Short-term use of NSAIDs or consult their GP
		Diuretics (e.g. bendroflumethiazide, furosemide, amiloride)	Hypertension	Short-term use of NSAIDs or consult their GP
		Methotrexate	Increased methotrexate toxicity	Consult patient's GP
		SSRIs (e.g. citalopram, fluoxetine)	Increased risk of bleeding	Short-term use of NSAIDs or consult their GP
Antibiotics	Penicillin-based antibiotics	Methotrexate	Increased risk of methotrexate toxicity with high dosages	Prescribe a lower dosage
		Warfarin	Can increase risk of bleeding (lower risk than other antibiotics)	Patients should be advised to be vigilant to increased risk of bleeding
	Metronidazole	NSAIDs (e.g. ibuprofen)	Increased risk of bleeding	Use an alternative antibiotic
		Phenytoin	Effect of phenytoin can be increased	Use an alternative antibiotic
		Warfarin	Increased risk of bleeding	Use an alternative antibiotic
	Macrolide antibiotics (erythromycin, clindamycin)	CCBs (e.g. amiodipine, nifedipine)	Increased and prolonged hypotensive effect of CCBs	Use an alternative antibiotic
		Simvastatin	Increased chance of muscle toxicity	Use an alternative antibiotic
		Clopidogrel	Increased risk of bleeding	Use an alternative antibiotic
		Warfarin	Increased risk of bleeding	Use an alternative antibiotic

ACE, angiotensin converting enzyme; CCB, calcium channel blocker; NSAID, non-steroidal anti-inflammatory drug; SSRI, selective serotonin reuptake inhibitor.

Endodontology at a Glance. First Edition. Alix Davies, Federico Foschi and Shanon Patel. © 2019 John Wiley & Sons, Ltd. Published 2019 by John Wiley & Sons, Ltd.
Companion website: www.wiley.com/go/davies/endodontology

Life expectancy is increasing and dentists will consequentially spend a greater amount of time treating older patients. Many of these patients will have retained a good proportion of their natural teeth, and would wish to retain them for as long as possible. Older patients present a variety of challenges which include more complex medical and social management factors as well as teeth that have been compromised with large restorations, cracks or root caries. Every case must be considered individually by assessing the strategic importance, restorability and periodontal health of the tooth, as well as the patient's wishes, to determine the most suitable management plan.

Medical history

Older patients often present with complex medical histories and it is important that medical history questionnaires are updated at each appointment. These patients can have cardiovascular, respiratory and central nervous system disorders and be taking medications that interact with antibiotics, analgesics or anaesthetics during dental treatment (Table 28.1). Liver and renal function may be reduced and consequently affect decisions on drug types and dosages that are administered during the dental procedure. Older patients are more likely to have been prescribed intravenous bisphosphonates. Extractions should be avoided in these patients and it may consequently be necessary to attempt root canal treatment in teeth that have a questionable restorability. Pacemakers are also common and can interact with older electric pulp testers, electosurgery equipment and some ultrasonics. A cardiologist's opinion would be wise prior to using such equipment. Type 2 diabetes is more prevalent in older patients and appointments should be planned to ensure that meals are not delayed or missed, which could otherwise result in hypoglycaemia.

Social factors

An elderly patient often relies on friends or relatives for transport to the surgery and may therefore wish to minimise the number of visits and complete as much as possible in one session. Other patients find that extended sessions in the chair are uncomfortable and would wish treatment to be spread out over shorter appointments. A neck support and mouth prop can help increase patient comfort. However, this cohort of patients are often less nervous and more tolerant of dental treatment than many of their younger counterparts.

Valid consent must be gained from all patients prior to elective treatment. If a patient has reduced mental capacity, a best interest meeting with physicians and relatives may be required.

Diagnosis and management of the older dentition

A full clinical and radiographic examination is required for endodontic diagnosis (see Chapters 4–7). Pulp testing can produce a greater number of false negative responses because of large restorations and pulp recession and canal sclerosis. Whilst cracked teeth and tooth discoloration are useful diagnostic indicators in younger patients, the older patient can have cracks in the majority of their teeth as well as a generalised yellow discoloration. Periodontal bone loss increases with age and there can be an increased number of lesions with a secondary endodontic or periodontal component. These teeth can require both endodontic and periodontal treatment and their prognosis is decreased.

Teeth are likely to be heavily restored and often posterior teeth are crowned. They can also exhibit root caries and tooth wear. A lone standing tooth is a common finding and is sometimes required to serve as an abutment for a bridge or denture. This could increase its risk of fracture. Patients requiring root canal retreatment may need removal of outdated root filling materials such as silver points and paste fillers (see Chapter 17).

Pulp capping procedures have a poor prognosis in elderly patients because of reduced pulpal blood supply. If the pulp is exposed during dental procedures, root canal treatment is therefore indicated. The blood supply to the apex of the tooth is also reduced and healing can occur at a slower rate. In immunocompromised elderly patients, the chances of postoperative flare up are higher. As a result of slower bone metabolism it is sometimes necessary to extend the postoperative review period prior to radiographically assessing healing of periapical lesions.

With increased age, cementum is laid down apically and therefore the cement–dentinal junction (CEJ) is further from the radiographic apex than it would be in a similar tooth of a younger patient (Figure 28.1). A root filling that is correctly placed to the position of the CEJ can consequently appear slightly short on the radiograph.

Secondary dentine deposition continues throughout life, causing recession of the pulp chamber and sclerosis of the canals. However, the calcifications are usually concentric and linear, and, once located, can usually be fully instrumented. This contrasts to cases of trauma or caries in a younger pulp that cause irregular tertiary dentine deposition and complete canal obliteration. The intraoral X-ray can overestimate the level of calcification of the canals, which becomes apparent under optimal illumination and magnification. Advanced radiographic imaging with CBCT can provide further evidence of the canal presence in doubtful cases.

Even in the presence of extremely calcified canals, the main lumen will harbour millions of bacteria. Each canal requires full chemomechanical preparation and obturation. Magnification, transillumination and careful examination of colour changes on the pulp floor are necessary to safely locate the root canals. Other techniques for finding the canals include the sodium hypochlorite bubble test, staining the pulp chamber floor with 1% methylene blue dye and searching for canal bleeding points. Once found, the canal should be flared and a crown down technique should be adopted with fine files and plenty of irrigant. Use of size 6 flexofiles or c-files may be indicated. Shorter files (21 mm length) can provide a better tactile feedback to progress in calcified canals. The use of abundant EDTA, both in liquid and gel form, can facilitate negotiation of the calcified canals.

If the canals cannot be found in a tooth with a periapical area, dentine should be gradually removed using fine ultrasonic tips under magnification. Radiographs should also be taken as apical progress is made to ensure that progression is in the correct plane and to reduce the risk of perforation. If the canal still cannot be located, root end surgery may be necessary.

29 Retain or replace?

Table 29.1 Comparison of studies assessing outcome for root canal treatment and replacement.

Root canal treatment	Prosthesis placement
Most studies examining primary root canal treatments assess cases performed by undergraduates or general dentists. Retreatment and surgical studies are usually performed by postgraduates and specialists	The majority of studies assess treatments provided by postgraduates or specialists
Success is measured against strict criteria. Evidence of healing of lesions is required rather than just survival in the mouth	Studies usually assess survival of the prosthesis – a prosthesis that has had complications is still often considered successful if it is retained in the mouth
There are often no strict entry criteria for root canal treatment studies	There are often extensive inclusion criteria. Patients may be excluded if they show parafunction, have diabetes, are smokers, have active infection or inadequate bone
Root canal treatments are commonly performed in areas with periapical infection and therefore a healing response is required	Prostheses are usually placed in disease-free areas and so do not require the same healing response

Figure 29.1 Strict criteria for endodontic success.

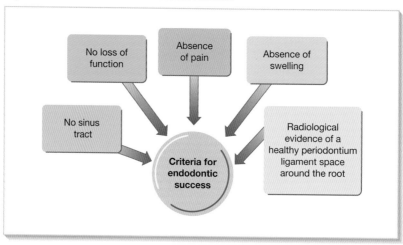

Figure 29.2 Complications encountered with prosthetic replacements.

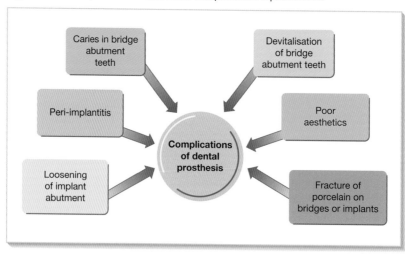

Endodontology at a Glance. First Edition. Alix Davies, Federico Foschi and Shanon Patel. © 2019 John Wiley & Sons, Ltd. Published 2019 by John Wiley & Sons, Ltd.
Companion website: www.wiley.com/go/davies/endodontology

When a tooth has pulpal or periapical pathology, the clinician must decide whether the tooth should be retained with endodontic therapy, or extracted and, if necessary, replaced. The options for replacement include an implant supported crown, bridge or denture. The dentist should discuss each suitable option with the patient, describing the procedures along with advantages, disadvantages, required time and costs for each. This enables the patient to make an informed decision about their treatment.

Both root canal treatment and placement of a prosthesis aim to provide an aesthetic functional unit that can withstand masticatory forces. Root canal treatment includes non-surgical primary treatments, retreatments or root end surgery. It aims to retain the tooth whilst an implant, bridge or denture replaces the missing tooth.

Comparison of the outcomes between different procedures

It is often difficult to directly compare the success rates of procedures such as implants with root canal treatments as study designs and success criteria are different (Table 29.1). Endodontic treatment outcome is usually determined by strict criteria (Figure 29.1) with success rates varying between 60% and 100% (see Chapter 22). Surgery traditionally had a very low success rate but microsurgery for appropriate patients now produces healing in over 90% of cases (see Chapter 23). However, if survival of the tooth in the mouth rather than healing of the lesion is assessed, over 95% of root treated teeth are retained at least 4–8 years postoperatively. The main reason for extraction is coronal tooth fracture in the absence of a cuspal coverage restoration. These survival rates compare favourably to prostheses replacement where single unit implants and conventional bridges both have a 95% survival. However, the prostheses still develop technical, biological and aesthetic complications (Figure 29.2). Adhesive bridges originally had a lower survival rate than conventional bridges but they have become more predictable with maximal coverage designs and improved resin cements.

Whilst the overall outcomes for root canal treatment and replacement prostheses are very similar, certain factors affect the prognosis of each. Therefore, each case must be considered individually to determine the most suitable option for the patient.

Factors for consideration when deciding whether to retain or replace a tooth

1 **Medical history;** Patients taking IV bisphosphonates are not suitable candidates for extraction and therefore these teeth should be retained if possible. Diabetes decreases the success rate of endodontic treatment and implant placement but is considered a complication rather than a contraindication. Smoking adversely affects the prognosis of root canal treatment and implant placement.

2 **Restorability of tooth;** The amount of remaining tooth tissue must be assessed to ensure there is enough for a ferrule. Any teeth that have cracks extending below the gingivae, or into the root canals, are not suitable for root canal treatment.

3 **Periodontal status;** Teeth with periodontal and endodontic involvement have a lower survival rate. However, implant placement in patients with periodontal disease is associated with an increased risk of developing peri-implant mucositis or implantitis. Bridges and dentures are also often not ideal because of poor abutment support. There can be many teeth with a poor prognosis if the periodontal disease is generalised and therefore it is necessary to consider the dentition as a whole rather than focus on one individual tooth during treatment planning.

4 **Amount and quality of alveolar bone;** It is important that the quality and quantity of bone, and the proximity of vital structures, are assessed when considering implant placement. Bone grafting can be required. Bony defects and extensive alveolar resorption are difficult to mask with bridges and so a denture may be more suitable.

5 **Status of adjacent teeth;** Fixed conventional bridge preparations irreversibly destroy abutment tooth tissue, increasing the risk of pulp necrosis. Conversely, adhesive bridges involve no tooth preparation. However, they rely on the abutment tooth being minimally restored. Root treated teeth are not ideal abutments because of their reduced stiffness. If a tooth cannot be retained with root canal therapy, implants are often a preferable solution, as they do not damage the abutment teeth.

6 **Parafunction;** Bruxism can increase the risk of fracture or loss of a restoration, whether it is a crown, a root treated tooth or implant. Patients should be provided with occlusal appliances to reduce the risk of mechanical failure.

7 **Aesthetics;** Retaining the natural tooth preserves the gingival contour. Bleaching, direct composite veneers and indirect restorations can improve the appearance of a root filled tooth. Implants and bridges can provide a good aesthetic result but it can be difficult to reproduce the natural gingival contour.

8 **Individual patient factors and wishes;** Patient anxiety and cooperation, gag reflexes, mouth opening and financial constraints are factors that require consideration. Implants are contraindicated in children and it is important to retain their teeth for as long as possible with endodontic treatment unless extractions can be incorporated into an orthodontic treatment plan.

Both root canal treatment and replacement with a prosthesis can have high success rates when performed correctly. However, with the exception of extraction and no replacement, no treatment option carries a lifetime guarantee and it is necessary to plan for failure. In many cases, it would therefore be prudent to perform the least destructive option of root canal treatment first. Should endodontic treatment fail, the patient has a variety of options available to them. However, dental heroics on unrestorable teeth are no longer necessary, as other options can provide a more predictable result.

30 Teeth whitening

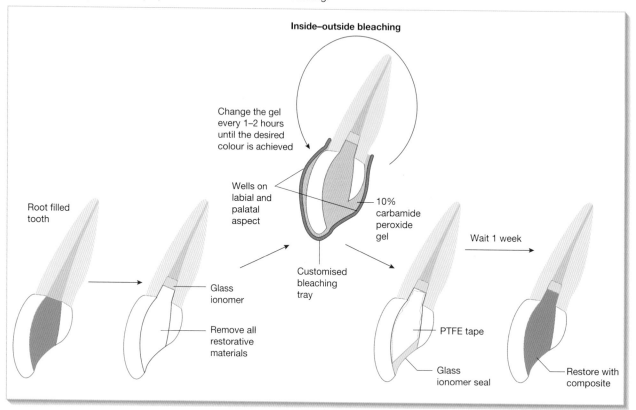

Figure 30.1 Stages of tooth preparation for non-vital tooth bleaching.

Inside–outside bleaching

Change the gel every 1–2 hours until the desired colour is achieved

Wells on labial and palatal aspect

10% carbamide peroxide gel

Wait 1 week

Root filled tooth

Glass ionomer

Remove all restorative materials

Customised bleaching tray

PTFE tape

Glass ionomer seal

Restore with composite

Box 30.1 Causes of extrinsic discoloration.

- Foods — Berries
  Tomato sauce
- Drinks — Tea
  Coffee
  Red wine
- Cigarettes — Tar
  Nicotine
- Mouthwashes — Chlorhexidine

Box 30.2 Contraindications for tooth bleaching.

- Severe root resorption
- Very sensitive teeth
- Leaking restorations
- Extremely dark stains may not be affected by tooth whitening
- Patients with leukoplakia or lichen planus as it can increase gingival aggravation

Causes of tooth discoloration

Extrinsic stains are superficial stains that usually occur following deposition of pigmented substances on the enamel surface. This accumulation is greater in patients with poor oral hygiene, smokers and those who ingest certain foods and beverages (Box 30.1). The pigments are retained as a result of interactions with the enamel pellicle that is adsorbed on to the enamel surface.

Intrinsic stains are deeper and caused by a variety of inherited and acquired factors. Amelogenesis imperfecta, dentinogenesis imperfecta and ingestion of excessive fluoride adversely affects the calcification of enamel, resulting in discoloration. Drugs such as tetracycline are oxidised to produce pigmented molecules that become incorporated into the dentine. Ageing causes the teeth to appear darker because of the production of secondary dentine that is more opaque and yellow than primary dentine. Tooth wear reduces the thickness of enamel, allowing the more darkly coloured dentine to dominate. Other causes of intrinsic staining include dental decay, bacterial pigments, release of metals from dental restorative materials and release of blood pigments in patients with pulpal damage.

Mechanism of tooth bleaching

Tooth whitening uses agents such as hydrogen peroxide, or its precursor carbamide peroxide. They diffuse through the enamel and dentine and dissociate to produce unstable free radicals. The radicals interact with double bonds of organic pigments, breaking them into smaller molecules of a different configuration. These changes alter the absorption and reflective properties of the tooth, producing a lighter appearance.

Methods of tooth bleaching

Whitening of teeth with an intact nerve supply is known as vital tooth bleaching. This includes 'in surgery' bleaching, dentist supervised 'take home' bleaching and supply of over-the-counter products.

Non-vital bleaching is performed on root treated teeth and includes 'inside outside' bleaching and the 'walking' bleach techniques.

Bleaching is a safe aesthetic technique that is conservative and cost effective compared with alternative methods of improving appearance such as crowns and veneers. Contraindications to bleaching are shown in Box 30.2.

In surgery bleaching

This method is performed in the dental chair. The soft tissues are retracted and rubber or paint-on gingival dam should be positioned to isolate the teeth and protect the gingivae. Gel (25–40% hydrogen peroxide) is then applied to the selected tooth surfaces. It is activated with heat or light to increase the dissociation of hydrogen peroxide. The gel can be washed off after a set time period and new gel applied until the desired appearance is reached. The lightening effect is immediate and the dentist has control over the shade. There is no reliance on patient compliance to wear bleaching trays. However, the bleach is caustic and therefore meticulous preparation of the area is essential to avoid soft tissue burns. Isolation of the teeth is time consuming and the surgery time required results in treatment being expensive. The teeth become dehydrated during the procedure and will therefore appear lighter immediately after treatment. Some patients notice regression of the shade in the hours and days after treatment.

Nightguard vital bleaching

External bleaching uses 10–20% carbamide peroxide (3–6% hydrogen peroxide) that is placed in wells in a customised tray. Patients should wear this for 8 hours in a 24-hour period. Most will wear it overnight for at least 2 weeks. It is a cheaper technique involving less chairside time. There are minimal adverse effects and the shade can be controlled by the patient. Transient thermal sensitivity is a common side effect although this will cease once treatment has finished. It does not usually affect the patient's ability to complete the course of treatment. Nightguard vital bleaching does not interfere with the health of the pulp or the microhardness of the teeth. However, it relies on patient compliance and some are unable to tolerate the trays or the metallic taste of the bleach.

Over-the-counter products

These products comprise gum shields, strips and whitening toothpastes. Care must be taken when choosing these products, as they are not all US Food and Drug Administration (FDA) approved. The concentration of the active ingredients is not always high enough for the product to be effective and, as the product is not held in a customised tray, it may fit poorly. This results in leakage of the gels, causing blistering and sensitivity. The 'wash out' from the tray dilutes the remaining gel, reducing its effectiveness.

Non-vital tooth bleaching

Inside–outside bleaching

This method of bleaching is used in a healthy asymptomatic root filled tooth. An impression should be taken and a tray constructed with labial and palatal wells. All the restorative material should be removed from the access cavity and the coronal part of the root filling should be cut to 2–3 mm below the cervical level. A thin layer of glass ionomer cement can be placed over the root filling, leaving the access cavity unfilled (Figure 30.1). Carbamide peroxide 10% gel should be injected from the syringe into the access cavity, and also placed in the wells of the tray prior to its insertion into the mouth. The gel should be refreshed every 1–2 hours. The patient often achieves their desired whitening effect within a few days.

Walking bleach technique

The tooth is prepared as for inside–outside bleaching and then a mixture of sodium perborate crystals and water are sealed into the pulp chamber. This should be changed every 7–10 days until the desired shade is reached.

Definitive composite restorations should be delayed for a week after bleaching is complete, as the hydrogen peroxide will inhibit polymerisation of the composite.

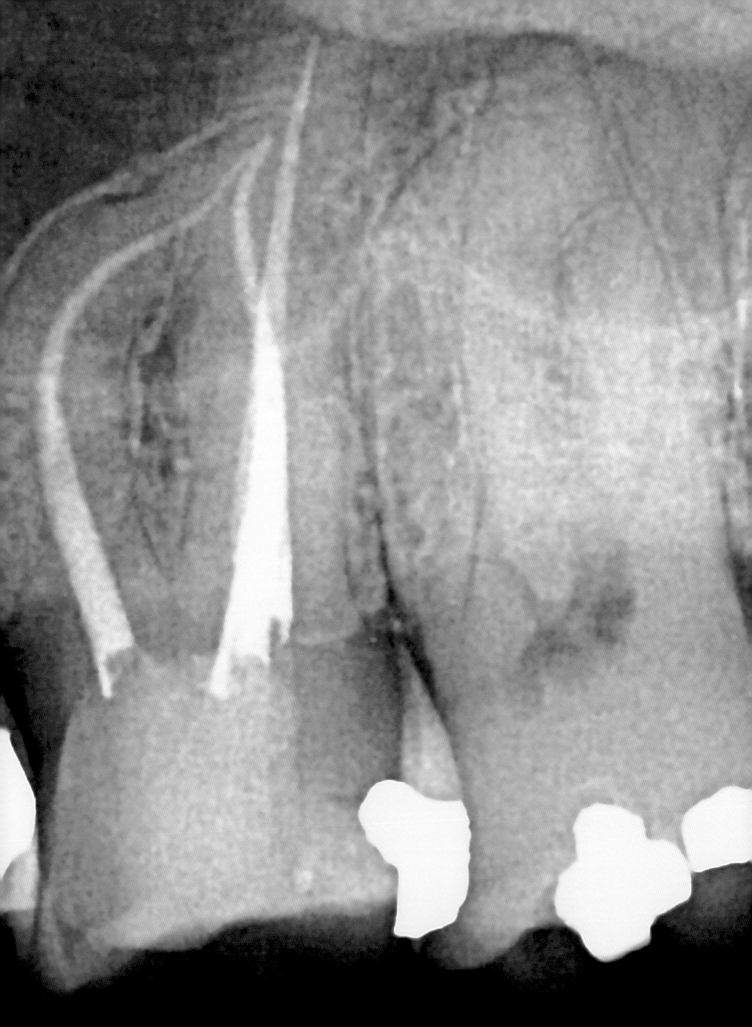

Trauma

Part 7

Chapters

31 Assessment of traumatic injuries

Figure 31.1 (a) The relative ages at which children have traumatic episodes. (b) The gender disparity in dental trauma experienced by children and adolescents.

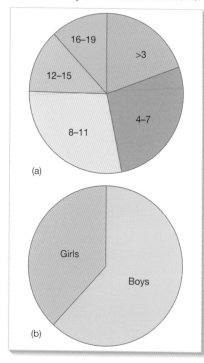

(a)

(b)

Figure 31.2 (a) The relative incidence of tooth fracture injuries. (b) The relative incidence of luxation injuries.

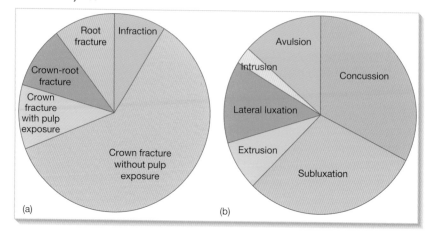

(a)

(b)

Figure 31.3 A diagram can be used in the patient notes to show clearly the position of traumatic injuries.

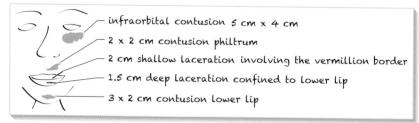

infraorbital contusion 5 cm x 4 cm

2 x 2 cm contusion philtrum

2 cm shallow laceration involving the vermillion border

1.5 cm deep laceration confined to lower lip

3 x 2 cm contusion lower lip

Figure 31.4 This patient had trauma to his UR1 and UL1 which were both extirpated prior to referral for assessment of possible fractures. Periapical radiographs at different angulations show a fracture to be evident on the UR1. However, it is not possible to identify if there is one or more fracture, and the proximity of the fragments to each other.

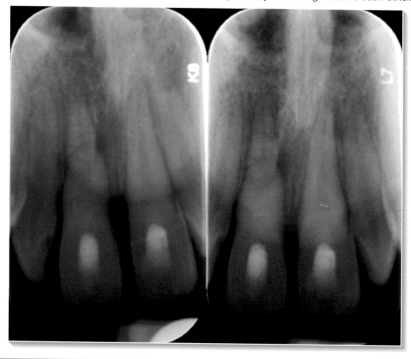

Figure 31.5 The CBCT reconstructed images provide more definitive information about the UR1 root fracture and surrounding bone.

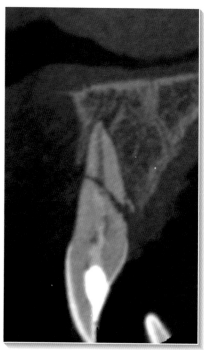

Endodontology at a Glance. First Edition. Alix Davies, Federico Foschi and Shanon Patel. © 2019 John Wiley & Sons, Ltd. Published 2019 by John Wiley & Sons, Ltd.
Companion website: www.wiley.com/go/davies/endodontology

Dental trauma affects all age groups but most commonly occurs in children (Figure 31.1). Trauma usually affects the maxillary incisors. Dental injuries involve fractures or luxations of the teeth (Figure 31.2). One-third of injuries show a combination of both. When a patient presents after a traumatic episode, a full history and systematic clinical examination are required, irrespective of the apparent severity of the injury. This facilitates more appropriate management and reduces the risk of missing injuries that are not immediately apparent.

History

• The medical history may reveal allergies, bleeding disorders or other conditions that could influence subsequent treatment decisions.
• The tetanus status of the patient should be established.
• A dental history includes previous traumatic episodes and treatment provided. This information assists in explaining radiographic findings such as the cessation in root development, apical pathology or obliteration of the pulp canals.

Detailed information is required relating to the current injury – this should be carefully documented as it can have future legal implications for the patient. Questioning should include the following:
• Where did the patient sustain the injury?
• When did the patient sustain the injury?
• How did the injury occur?
• Did the patient lose consciousness?
• Has the patient already had treatment elsewhere?
• If there are missing tooth fragments or teeth, have they been accounted for?
• Is there any disturbance in the patient's bite?
• Are any teeth sore to touch or bite with?
• Are any teeth particularly painful or sensitive to hot, cold or sweet sensations?

If there was an extended period of unconsciousness or the patient presents with amnesia, nausea or vomiting the patient should be referred for immediate medical attention.

If there is uncertainty regarding the whereabouts of any portion of the tooth, referral for a chest radiograph may be indicated to ensure the fragment was not inhaled.

The patient should have his/her face and mouth cleaned with water or saline prior to the clinical examination. This improves the patient's comfort and allows a more thorough assessment of any injuries.

Extraoral examination

The patient should be examined for any contusions, lacerations or facial asymmetry. Diagrams in the notes can be helpful to show the exact position and extent of the lesion (Figure 31.3).

The mandible, maxillary, infraorbital and zygomatic regions should be palpated to assess any tenderness and deformities that indicate skeletal fractures. Jaw opening should also be assessed with any clicks or deviations noted.

The lips should be examined for lacerations or contusions; these should be palpated to assess for embedded tooth fragments. However, the oral musculature often contracts tightly around foreign bodies making it difficult to identify deeply embedded fragments.
• Intraoral examination involves a soft tissue examination for sublingual haemorrhages and lacerations that can indicate underlying jaw fractures.
• The occlusion should be assessed and any fractured crowns, abnormalities in tooth position or tooth mobility should be documented.
• The teeth in the area of the trauma should be percussed to assess for tenderness.
• Pulp sensitivity testing with an electronic pulp tester and Endofrost should be performed and recorded as baseline readings. Laser Doppler monitors can be used to assess pulpal blood flow if they are available, although this may be more relevant in follow-up appointments.

Clinical photography

Photographic images can be taken with the patient's consent. These provide an exact record of the traumatic injuries. and can be used to plan and monitor treatment and as well as to support legal claims.

Radiographic examination

Radiographic examination is required to assess the site of trauma. Multiple views can be necessary to enable visualisation of lateral luxations, root and alveolar fractures.

It may also be necessary to radiograph the soft tissues to assess and locate foreign bodies. A film should be placed between the lips and the dental arch and the exposure time should be reduced by 50%. If a foreign body is revealed, a lateral exposure can be necessary to locate the object.

Cone beam computed tomography (CBCT) is indicated when complex trauma (e.g. luxation, root fracture) or alveolar bone fracture is suspected. In addition to being a more comfortable procedure for the patient to tolerate, it will provide the clinician with enhanced images of the trauma site to improve management of the injury (Figures 31.4 and 31.5).

Referral

The prognosis of traumatised teeth is often dependent on the time interval between the traumatic episode and treatment (i.e. replantation, repositioning of teeth or pulp procedures). However, treatment should not be performed if this would delay more urgent medical attention. Patients with suspected jaw fractures should be appropriately referred to oral and maxillofacial units for management of these injuries.

32 Management of crown fractures

Figure 32.1 Partial and full pulpotomy procedures.

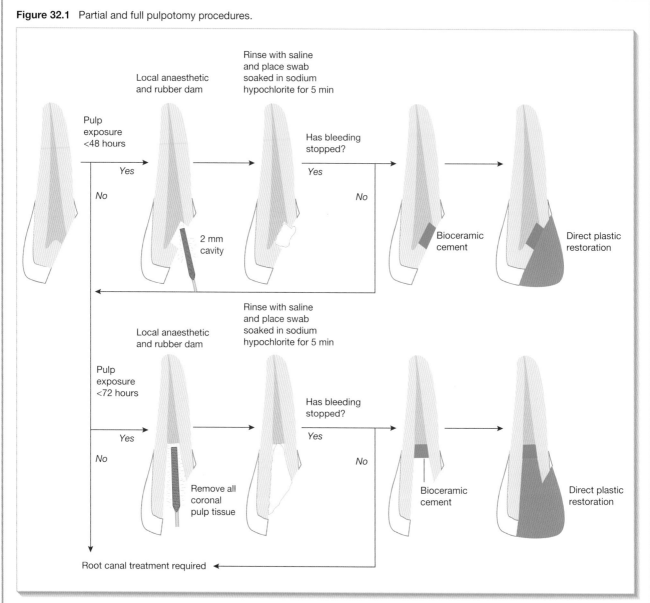

Table 32.1 Signs of fractures involving the crown of the tooth.

	Enamel infraction	Fracture within enamel	Fracture within enamel and dentine	Fracture involving the enamel, dentine and pulp
Visual examination	A crack is visible on the crown surface	Chip of tooth confined to enamel	Fracture involving enamel and dentine No pulp exposure evident	There is loss of the enamel and dentine and bleeding will be evident from the exposed pulp
Mobility	Normal	Normal	Normal	Normal
Percussion test	Not tender	Not tender	Not tender	Not tender
Pulp vitality testing	Normally positive	Normally positive	Normally positive	Normally positive
Radiographic examination	No radiographic abnormalities noticed	Loss of enamel, dentine layer in tact Periapical tissues healthy	Loss of enamel and dentine only Periapical tissues healthy	Loss of a larger amount of enamel and dentine Periapical tissues healthy

Endodontology at a Glance. First Edition. Alix Davies, Federico Foschi and Shanon Patel. © 2019 John Wiley & Sons, Ltd. Published 2019 by John Wiley & Sons, Ltd.
Companion website: www.wiley.com/go/davies/endodontology

Damage to the clinical crown can be in the form of an infraction, an uncomplicated or complicated coronal fracture. Examination and assessment of traumatic injuries are discussed in Chapter 31 and the diagnostic signs are shown in Table 32.1.

Infractions

• An infraction is a crack of the enamel with no loss of tooth structure.
• Management involves etching of the area and sealing with resin to prevent microleakage and possible future staining of the cracks.
• In teeth where this is the only injury, no follow-up is required.

Uncomplicated coronal fractures

An uncomplicated coronal fracture either involves just the enamel, or the enamel and dentine; there is no pulpal exposure. Management aims to restore the appearance of the tooth and reduce any sensitivity. It should also reduce microleakage by sealing the exposed dentinal tubules.

Calcium hydroxide can be placed as an indirect pulp cap if the fracture has occurred close to the pulp chamber. If the separated tooth fragment is available, it can be rebonded. Otherwise, glass ionomer cements can be placed as a provisional restoration or, if time permits, composite can be placed to restore the defect. Patients should be reviewed clinically and radiographically at 2 months and 1 year.

Complicated coronal fractures

Complicated crown fractures expose the enamel, dentine and pulp. Management depends on the stage of root development.

Immature teeth with open apices

It is important to preserve the vitality of the pulp in an immature tooth with an open apex as its necrosis would halt dentine development. This would result in a tooth with thin dentinal walls at high risk of future fracture. Performing root canal treatment on a tooth with an open apex is also complex and time consuming. Patient cooperation is necessary but can be difficult to attain when the patient is young. Vital pulp therapy should therefore be attempted whenever possible. Success is higher when treatment is performed within 48 hours of the injury. After this there is an increased risk of bacterial contamination which will continue to progress apically. Vital pulp therapy includes pulp capping, partial (Cvek) pulpotomy and full coronal pulpotomy.

Pulp capping

Direct pulp capping involves placing a Bioceramic material such as Biodentine or MTA directly on to the pulp exposure prior to restoring the crown with composite. However, it is not to be recommended, as immediately after trauma the exposed pulp becomes superficially inflamed. If this inflamed tissue is not removed, there is the risk of the inflammation progressing

apically. It is also difficult to produce a good coronal seal and future bacterial leakage is therefore possible. In the absence of additional luxation injuries, the success rate of this procedure is about 80%. The success of a partial pulpotomy is 95% and so the latter is therefore preferable.

Partial pulpotomy

Partial pulpotomy is the treatment of choice in pulps that have been exposed for less than 48 hours (Figure 32.1). After administration of local anaesthetic and rubber dam, the area should be disinfected with sodium hypochlorite. A 2-mm cavity is prepared into the pulp using a high speed handpiece and sterile diamond bur with copious water irrigation. If bleeding is excessive, it may be necessary to increase the depth of the preparation. The area should be rinsed with saline and then a cotton wool swab with sodium hypochlorite should be placed. This removes damaged pulp cells and dentine chips. It also controls the bleeding without injuring the healthy underlying pulp tissue. Once the bleeding has ceased, calcium hydroxide or white MTA can be placed in the pulpal cavity. This should be sealed with glass ionomer cement. Composite resin can then be placed to restore the defect.

Full pulpotomy

This is recommended in teeth where the pulp has been exposed for 48–72 hours. In addition, if there is excessive haemorrhage when attempting a partial pulpotomy, it may be necessary to increase the depth of the preparation to a full pulpotomy. The technique is the same as for the partial pulpotomy but the pulp is removed to the level of the root orifice.

Clinical and radiographic monitoring is required at 2 months and 1 year. Clinical monitoring involves vitality testing with the electric pulp tester and Endofrost as well as confirming absence of symptoms. However, a tooth that has undergone a full pulpotomy procedure has had the entire coronal pulp removed and it is therefore unlikely to respond to sensitivity tests. Radiographic monitoring becomes very important for these patients and will confirm that the root is continuing to develop and there is no periapical pathology.

Root canal treatment

This can be required if the pulp has been exposed for a considerable time, or vital pulp therapy has failed. A Bioceramic cement should be used to form an apical plug. Composite can also be placed in the coronal third of the root canal to improve its resistance to fracture (see Chapter 16).

Closed apices

Pulpotomy procedures can be attempted in older patients with closed apices if they present immediately for treatment. However, successful preservation of vitality is lower. As root formation is complete, maintenance of a vital pulp is not as important as for patients with immature open apices. Therefore, root canal treatment is often the treatment of choice. This can also be indicated if a post is considered necessary to restore the tooth.

33 Management of (crown-) root fractures

Figure 33.1 (a) Crown root fracture without pulpal involvement. (b) Crown root fracture with pulpal involvement. (c) Root fracture.

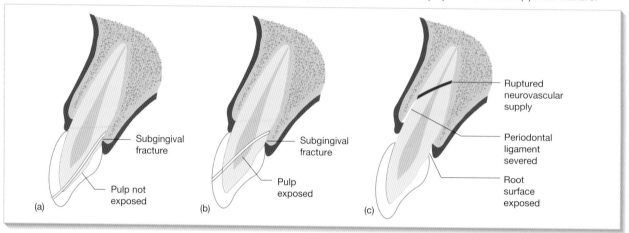

(a) Subgingival fracture / Pulp not exposed

(b) Subgingival fracture / Pulp exposed

(c) Ruptured neurovascular supply / Periodontal ligament severed / Root surface exposed

Figure 33.2 Various healing responses post root fracture.

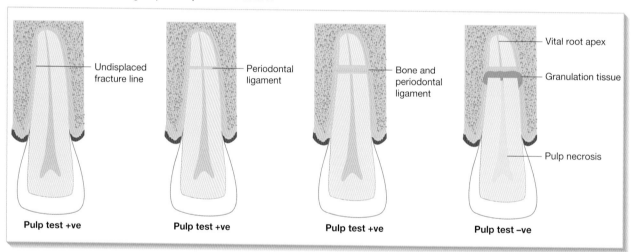

Undisplaced fracture line — Pulp test +ve

Periodontal ligament — Pulp test +ve

Bone and periodontal ligament — Pulp test +ve

Vital root apex / Granulation tissue / Pulp necrosis — Pulp test −ve

Table 33.1 Diagnostic signs of crown root and root fractures.

	Crown root fracture with no pulp involvement	Crown root fracture with pulp involvement	Root fracture
Visual examination	A crown fracture will be seen that extends below the gingival margin	A crown fracture will be seen that extends below the gingival margin	There can be bleeding from the gingival sulcus and the coronal segment can be displaced and positioned below the occlusal line of adjacent teeth
Mobility	The coronal fragment will be mobile	The coronal fragment will be mobile	The coronal fragment will be mobile
Percussion test	Tender	Tender	Tender
Pulp vitality testing	The apical portion usually responds positively to pulp testing	The apical portion usually responds positively to pulp testing	Pulp testing usually provides a negative response
Radiographic examination	The fracture line is often not visible	The fracture line is often not visible	A fracture line is visible, either in a horizontal or oblique plane

Endodontology at a Glance. First Edition. Alix Davies, Federico Foschi and Shanon Patel. © 2019 John Wiley & Sons, Ltd. Published 2019 by John Wiley & Sons, Ltd.
Companion website: www.wiley.com/go/davies/endodontology

Root fractures are confined to the root whilst crown root fractures involve the root and the crown of the tooth, with or without pulpal exposure. Examination and assessment of traumatic injuries are discussed in Chapter 31 and the diagnostic signs of root fractures are shown in Table 33.1.

Crown root fracture without pulpal involvement

• The tooth has fractured in a diagonal plane involving part of the enamel, dentine and cementum (Figure 33.1).

• Whilst radiographs may show part of the fracture, it is difficult to identify the apical extent and a CBCT scan is recommended to visualise the full fracture. However, this may not be available on site.

• The mobile fragment should be bonded to the remaining tooth tissue to improve comfort until imaging is performed and a definitive treatment plan has been made.

There are various management options, including removal of the mobile fragment, possibly with a gingivectomy, orthodontic or surgical extrusion of the tooth to coronally expose the entire fragment, decoronation or extraction of the tooth.

In the interim period between emergency and definitive treatment, and after the definitive treatment is performed, the patient should be recommended to adhere to a soft diet. They must be advised on the importance of good oral hygiene using a soft toothbrush. Chlorhexidine mouth rinses are also beneficial.

Crown root fracture with pulpal involvement

The tooth has fractured in a diagonal plane involving part of the enamel, dentine and cementum and additionally involving the pulp (Figure 33.1). A CBCT scan is again recommended to assess the extent of these fractures and emergency treatment to stabilise the fractured portion is performed until a full management plan has been decided. If the tooth has an open apex, a partial pulpotomy is recommended to preserve pulpal vitality (see Chapter 32). The loose fragment can be bonded to the remaining tooth tissue, or splinted to the adjacent teeth.

The options for management are the same as for crown root fractures without pulpal involvement. However, the teeth additionally require a pulpotomy or root canal treatment.

Root fracture

When root fracture occurs, the coronal segment is displaced coronally whilst the apical segment stays in situ (Figure 33.1).

There can be a single horizontal, oblique fracture, or multiple fractures. CBCT scans improve visualisation of the fractures but repositioning and splinting of the coronal segment should not be delayed by sending the patient for a scan if these facilities are not available on site.

Emergency treatment involves immediate repositioning of the displaced coronal fragment. A radiograph should be taken to ensure correct repositioning and the tooth should be stabilised with a flexible splint for 4 weeks. If the root fracture is in the cervical third, the splinting time may need to be increased up to 4 months. If the patient presents for treatment some time after the traumatic episode, it may not be possible to completely reapproximate the two segments and healing will be compromised. The patient should comply with a soft diet and good oral hygiene. Supplemental chlorhexidine mouth rinses are beneficial.

Clinical and radiographic reviews are required at 1 month (coinciding with splint removal), 2, 4 and 6 months and 1 year. Yearly reviews are then required for up to 5 years. One of the four responses to treatment will be evident (Figure 33.2):

Necrosis of the coronal segment occurs in about 25% cases. However, circulation to the apical portion is not disrupted and therefore necrosis of this portion is very rare. Root canal treatment is indicated if there is necrosis of the coronal segment and in most cases will involve instrumentation and obturation of the coronal portion to the position of the fracture. Bioceramic cements are recommended to create an apical plug at the fracture line. In the rare instance where the apical segment is necrotic and shows a periapical radiolucency, root canal treatment can be performed through the fracture line. However, this is very difficult to perform in the majority of cases where the fracture has not healed. Surgical removal of the apical segment provides a more predictable alternative.

Factors that influence the outcome of root fractured teeth include the degree of dislocation and mobility of the coronal segment. Immature teeth have a better prognosis than mature teeth because of the larger size of the apical opening in the coronal segment, therefore improved chance of revascularisation. Quality of treatment is important, with improved success rates demonstrated when treatment has not been delayed, the root segments have been closely approximated and correct splinting times have been chosen. Root fractures occuring within the cervical third have an equal prognosis to those fractures in the mid and apical thirds providing that the fracture occurs below the crest of the bone.

Maintaining a healthy periodontal status with no loss of attachment is of paramount importance to avoid progression of the infection from the periodontal to the endodontic compartment.

34 Management of luxation injuries

Figure 34.1 Various luxation injuries (a) Concussion, (b) Subluxation, (c) Lateral luxation, (d) Extrusive luxation, (e) Intrusive luxation.

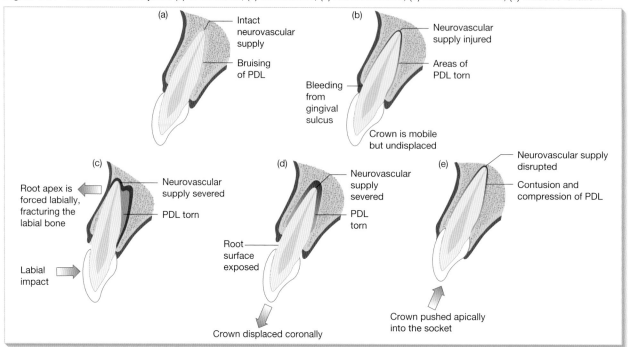

(a)
- Intact neurovascular supply
- Bruising of PDL

(b)
- Neurovascular supply injured
- Areas of PDL torn
- Bleeding from gingival sulcus
- Crown is mobile but undisplaced

(c)
- Root apex is forced labially, fracturing the labial bone
- Neurovascular supply severed
- PDL torn
- Labial impact

(d)
- Neurovascular supply severed
- PDL torn
- Root surface exposed
- Crown displaced coronally

(e)
- Neurovascular supply disrupted
- Contusion and compression of PDL
- Crown pushed apically into the socket

Table 34.1 Diagnostic signs for each type of luxation injury.

	Concussion	Subluxation	Lateral luxation	Extrusive luxation	Intrusive luxation
Visual examination	No displacement	No displacement	Crown is usually displaced in a palatal-lingual direction	Crown appears elongated and at a lower occlusal level than adjacent teeth	The crown appears shorter and at a higher occlusal level than the adjacent teeth. In severe intrusions it may not be visible
Mobility	Not increased	Slightly increased	Often immobile	Greatly increased	Immobile
Percussion test	Tender	Tender	Tender	Tender	Tender
Pulp vitality testing	Usually positive	50% will initially respond positively to pulp tests	Unless the displacement is minimal, the pulp test will usually provide a negative response	Unless the displacement is minimal, the pulp test will usually provide a negative response	Negative
Radiographic examination	The tooth is in the normal position	The tooth is in the normal position	A widened periodontal ligament space may be seen	A widened periodontal space will be seen at the apex	The periodontal ligament space may be absent around part, or all of the tooth. The cementum-enamel junction is at a higher level than adjacent teeth

Table 34.2 Splinting times for luxation injuries.

Dental injury	Splinting time
Subluxation	2 weeks (if necessary at all)
Lateral luxation	4 weeks
Extrusion	2 weeks
Intrusion	4 weeks
Root fracture	4 weeks (unless fracture is at the cervical margin where it may be necessary to splint for up to 4 months)
Alveolar bone fracture	4 weeks

Endodontology at a Glance. First Edition. Alix Davies, Federico Foschi and Shanon Patel. © 2019 John Wiley & Sons, Ltd. Published 2019 by John Wiley & Sons, Ltd.
Companion website: www.wiley.com/go/davies/endodontology

Luxation injuries account for 30–40% of dental injuries. They include concussion, subluxation, lateral luxation, extrusive luxation and intrusive luxation. Examination and assessment of traumatic injuries have been discussed in Chapter 31 and the diagnostic signs of each type of luxation are shown in Table 34.1.

Luxation injuries damage the periodontal ligament, cementum and alveolar bone. Healing of these tissues can be favourable if the injury is localised and mild. When the damage is more extensive, the prognosis is worse and the teeth are at an increased risk of resorption (see Chapter 3). There can also be damage to the neurovascular supply to the pulp. Revascularisation is possible in mild injuries and teeth with open apices, although pulp canal obliteration is a common finding. Pulp necrosis commonly occurs in more severe traumatic episodes, especially in lateral luxation and intrusion injuries. The canal will become infected if root canal treatment is not initiated. Management of luxation injuries aims to reposition the tooth to facilitate pulpal and periodontal healing. The tooth requires regular reviews and endodontic therapy may be required to prevent resorption and prolong the survival of the tooth. Referral to an Endodontist should be considered.

Concussion and subluxation

Concussion involves the bruising of supporting dental tissues. However, the neurovascular supply usually remains intact and, although there may be minor bleeding in the periodontal ligament, most areas remain healthy (Figure 34.1a). Subluxation injuries demonstrate slight loosening of the tooth coupled with reversible damage to the periodontal ligament and neurovascular supply (Figure 34.1b).

- No immediate treatment is usually required.
- Baseline pulp testing should be performed.
- If necessary, a flexible splint can be used to stabilise the teeth and increase comfort. However, it should be removed after 2 weeks.
- Patients should be advised on good oral hygiene techniques, chlorhexidine mouth rinses and a soft diet.
- Patients should be reviewed clinically and radiographically at 1 month, 2 months and 1 year.

Lateral luxation

A lateral luxation involves the displacement of the tooth in any direction other than axial. Usually, the crown is displaced palatally with the root moving labially where it may become entrapped in the bone. This is likely to cause disruption of the neurovascular supply and extensive injury to the periodontal ligament. There is often the additional complication of an alveolar bone fracture (Figure 34.1c).

- Emergency treatment should be performed under local anaesthetic where forceps or finger pressure can be used to disengage the apex and reposition the tooth.
- A flexible splint should be placed for 4 weeks (Table 34.2).

- Soft food, good oral hygiene and chlorhexidine rinses are recommended.
- The tooth must be reviewed clinically and radiographically after 1, 2 and 6 months, 1 year and then yearly for 5 years. This monitoring is essential to confirm revascularisation, otherwise infection and rapid inflammatory resorption can occur. Signs of revascularisation in a tooth with an open apex are the return of positive responses to vitality testing, radiographic signs of continuing root development and possible pulp obliteration.
- In a tooth with a closed apex, an absence of pulpal response after 3 months, with concomitant discoloration and radiographic signs of a periapical area, indicate an infected necrotic pulp. Root canal treatment is required.

Extrusive luxation

Extrusive luxation involves partial or complete tearing of the periodontal ligament, resulting in a degree of coronal displacement of the tooth. This can be accompanied by some lateral displacement. However, unlike lateral luxations, the alveolar bone remains intact (Figure 34.1d). Management and follow-up is the same as for lateral luxations with the exception that the splint is only placed for 2 weeks as there is no alveolar fracture.

Intrusive luxation

This involves displacement of the tooth apically into the socket. There is extensive periodontal ligament injury and disruption of the neurovascular supply. Intrusive injuries are also accompanied by contusion and fracture of the alveolar bone (Figure 34.1e). The management plan will depend on the maturity of the tooth and the degree of the intrusion.

- Allowing spontaneous eruption can lead to fewer complications than orthodontic or surgical repositioning. However, re-eruption can take considerable time, and needs to be closely monitored.
- If no movement has occured after a few weeks, orthodontic or surgical repositioning must be initiated to prevent ankylosis of the tooth.
- Orthodontic extrusion is the most time consuming and costly option. It also requires extended patient cooperation. However, it is useful when the patient has delayed seeking treatment or spontaneous eruption has failed. Surgical repositioning is indicated in severe intrusive cases and it is preferable to perform this immediately after the trauma when the periodontal ligament has already been severed. If this is performed, a flexible splint should be applied for 4 weeks.
- Teeth with closed apices are unlikely to revascularise and therefore root canal treatment is recommended as soon as possible.
- Teeth with open apices should be clinically and radiographically monitored with reviews after 1, 2 and 6 months, 1 year and yearly for 5 years. A tooth that fails to revascularise and subsequently becomes infected requires root canal treatment to prevent inflammatory root resorption.

35 Management of avulsed teeth

Figure 35.1 Flow chart showing the immediate and long term management of an avulsed tooth.

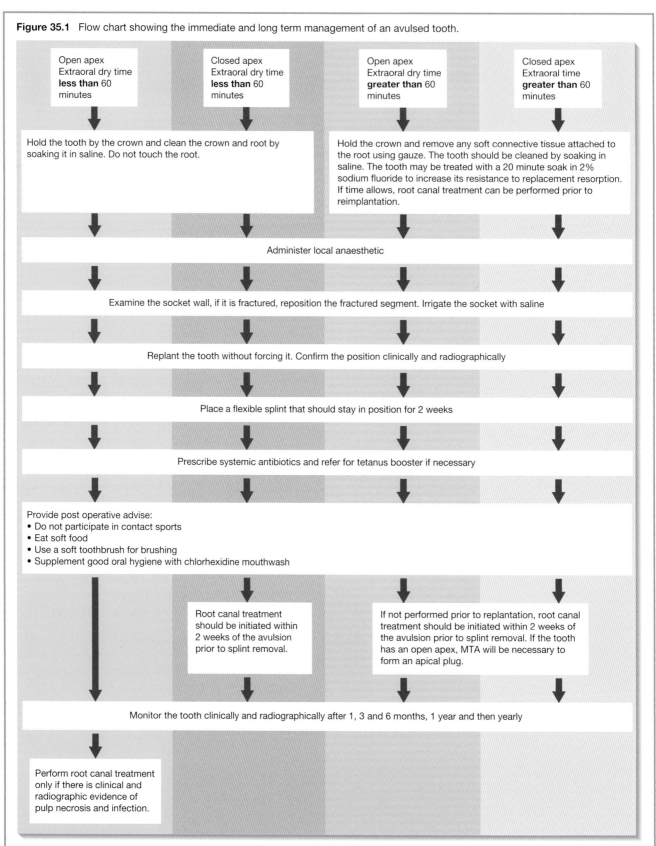

Open apex
Extraoral dry time
less than 60
minutes

Closed apex
Extraoral dry time
less than 60
minutes

Open apex
Extraoral dry time
greater than 60
minutes

Closed apex
Extraoral time
greater than 60
minutes

Hold the tooth by the crown and clean the crown and root by soaking it in saline. Do not touch the root.

Hold the crown and remove any soft connective tissue attached to the root using gauze. The tooth should be cleaned by soaking in saline. The tooth may be treated with a 20 minute soak in 2% sodium fluoride to increase its resistance to replacement resorption. If time allows, root canal treatment can be performed prior to reimplantation.

Administer local anaesthetic

Examine the socket wall, if it is fractured, reposition the fractured segment. Irrigate the socket with saline

Replant the tooth without forcing it. Confirm the position clinically and radiographically

Place a flexible splint that should stay in position for 2 weeks

Prescribe systemic antibiotics and refer for tetanus booster if necessary

Provide post operative advise:
• Do not participate in contact sports
• Eat soft food
• Use a soft toothbrush for brushing
• Supplement good oral hygiene with chlorhexidine mouthwash

Root canal treatment should be initiated within 2 weeks of the avulsion prior to splint removal.

If not performed prior to replantation, root canal treatment should be initiated within 2 weeks of the avulsion prior to splint removal. If the tooth has an open apex, MTA will be necessary to form an apical plug.

Monitor the tooth clinically and radiographically after 1, 3 and 6 months, 1 year and then yearly

Perform root canal treatment only if there is clinical and radiographic evidence of pulp necrosis and infection.

Endodontology at a Glance. First Edition. Alix Davies, Federico Foschi and Shanon Patel. © 2019 John Wiley & Sons, Ltd. Published 2019 by John Wiley & Sons, Ltd.
Companion website: www.wiley.com/go/davies/endodontology

An avulsion occurs when a tooth is fully displaced from its socket. The consequences of this are severance of the neurovascular supply to the pulp and tearing of the entire periodontal ligament. The outer cementum layer becomes exposed and is at high risk of desiccation and bacterial contamination.

Factors affecting the prognosis of avulsed teeth

An avulsed permanent tooth is one of the few emergency situations requiring immediate dental management. Several factors affect the prognosis of the tooth:

1 Time the tooth is out of the socket The shorter the time period between avulsion and replacement of the tooth in the socket, the better the prognosis. A short extraoral time increases the chance of revascularisation in teeth with an open apex. It also decreases the risk of resorption.

2 Storage medium Storing a tooth dry severely damages any viable cementum and periodontal ligament cells. Therefore, if the tooth cannot be reimplanted immediately, it should be placed in a storage medium. Milk, saliva and saline are suitable but water should be avoided as it is hypotonic and causes cell lysis. Chlorhexidine should also be avoided.

3 Splinting technique and time Flexible splinting for 2 weeks is recommended. Longer splinting times increase the risk of replacement resorption.

4 Condition of the alveolar bone Additional complications of alveolar bone fractures make repositioning of the tooth more difficult and decrease the prognosis of the tooth.

5 Stage of root development Teeth with open apices have a greater chance of revascularisation, but are also at higher risk of rapid internal or external inflammatory resorption or external replacement resorption.

Reimplantation is the treatment of choice for avulsed permanent teeth, even when a combination of unfavourable influences indicate the tooth would have a low chance of survival. The success of even a small percentage of cases make it worth giving each tooth a chance.

Avulsions most frequently occur in the 8–12 year age group. The subsequent eruption of the canine teeth results in undesirable tooth movements and centreline shifts if an upper incisor is missing. Even if the reimplanted tooth only lasts for a few years, its role as a space maintainer is invaluable. This can prevent protracted orthodontic treatment and the need to wear a removable appliance.

Failure to reimplant the tooth can cause dramatic horizontal and vertical tooth loss that can necessitate future costly and unpredictable bone augmentation procedures. In addition, the loss of a tooth can be physiologically stressful for the patient (and parents). Reimplantation eases the shock at this point and allows time to plan for a future replacement.

Providing emergency advice by phone

Emergency instructions should be given by phone, advising the patient, parent or other person present to:
• Find the tooth and hold it by the crown part only.

• It should be washed under running water for 10 seconds if it is dirty and replaced in the socket if possible. The patient should then bite on a handkerchief to keep it in position.
• If reimplantion is not possible, advice on suitable storage media should be given and the patient advised to see a dentist immediately.
• On attendance at the practice, the tooth should be left in situ whilst the area is cleansed. Clinical and radiographic examinations are necessary to confirm that the tooth has been repositioned correctly and any adjustments made.
• The tooth should be splinted with a flexible splint for 2 weeks, antibiotics prescribed and postoperative instructions given (Figure 35.1). Referral to an Endodontist should be considered.
• Mature teeth with closed apices will not revascularise and root canal treatment should therefore be initiated within 2 weeks of the traumatic episode.
• If the tooth has an open apex, root canal treatment should be initially avoided to allow for continued root development. Failure of revascularisation can make root canal treatment necessary in the future.
• Signs and symptoms suggestive of this include pain, tenderness on biting and long-term discoloration of the crown. Development of swelling or a sinus tract or radiographic evidence of a periapical radiolucency coupled with failure of continued root development indicate the need for endodontic intervention.

Reimplantation of the avulsed tooth in the dental surgery

If a patient presents with an avulsed tooth that has not been replaced, the flow diagram in Figure 35.1 should be followed.

Use of antibiotics

Systemic antibiotics are advised after an avulsed tooth has been replanted. Whilst tetracyclines such as doxycycline are recommended, they are contraindicated in some countries if children are under 12 years. Amoxicillin is an alternative.

Long-term follow-up

If a reimplanted tooth subsequently develops internal or external resorption, implants can be planned, but are only suitable once the patient completes her/his growth (at least 22 years of age). Therefore, all efforts must be concentrated into trying to maintain the tooth and alveolar bone until this point.

Replacement resorption (ankylosis) is the pathological fusion of the cementum or dentine to the alveolar bone (see Chapter 3). It can occur rapidly in preadolescents and can alter the local alveolar growth. This results in the apparent submergence of the tooth with associated functional and aesthetic defects. It is imperative therefore that these patients are followed up and, if submergence is noted, an appropriate referral made for decoronation of the crown. This facilitates submergence of the root, enabling the bony profile to be maintained.

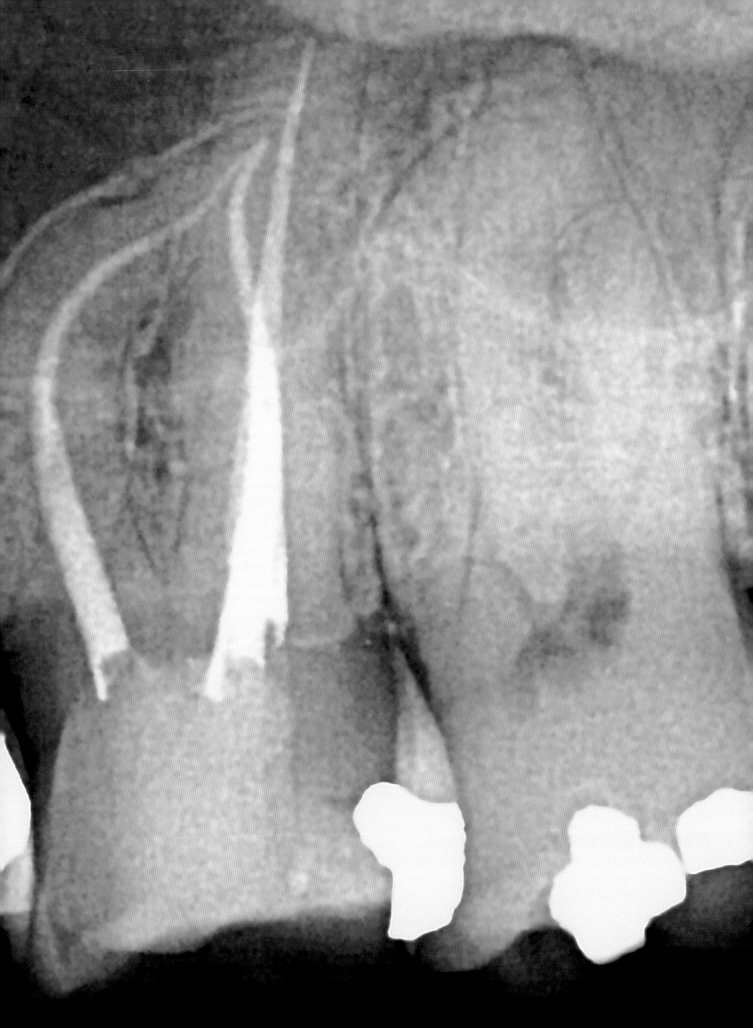

Risk management

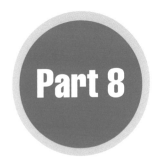

Part 8

Chapter

36 Risk management in endodontics

Figure 36.1 (a) Periapical radiograph showing a fractured spiral root filler in an UL4. The canal had not been disinfected prior to fracture and has been poorly obturated resulting in persistent chronic apical periodontitis. (b) Periapical radiograph showing a fractured file in the mesial root of LL6. The canal had been disinfected prior to instrument fracture at the apex, and the canal has been well obturated. This case is therefore likely to be successful.

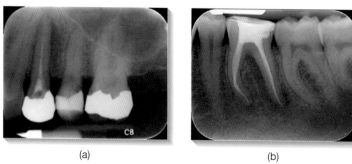

(a)   (b)

Figure 36.2 (a) Radiograph showing a perforation at the gingival margin when performing an access cavity on LL6. (b) Radiograph showing a strip perforation when instrumenting the LL6 distal root. (c) Radiograph showing a perforation on UL4 mesial aspect when placing a post.

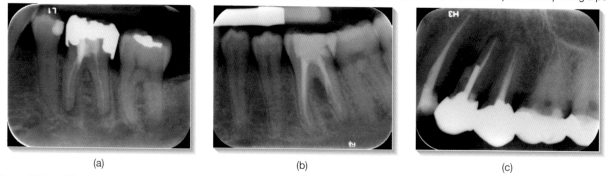

(a)   (b)   (c)

Figure 36.3 (a) Periapical radiograph showing LL6 with an extruded root filling in the mesial and distal canals. The patient subsequently developed pain and paraesthesia on her left lip and around the teeth on the lower left side. The reconstructed CBCT images show the root fillings terminating in the inferior dental canal. (b) Radiograph showing a canal where root filling was extruded. However, the canal had been thoroughly disinfected and well obturated. One year review shows the patient to be asymptomatic and there is periapical healing. (c) Periapical radiograph showing a short poorly condensed root filling on a LR6 that had periapical areas associated with the mesial and distal roots. (d) Periapical radiograph showing a root filled UL6 with silver points in the mesial and distal canals. (e) Periapical radiograph showing LL6 filled with a resin cement.

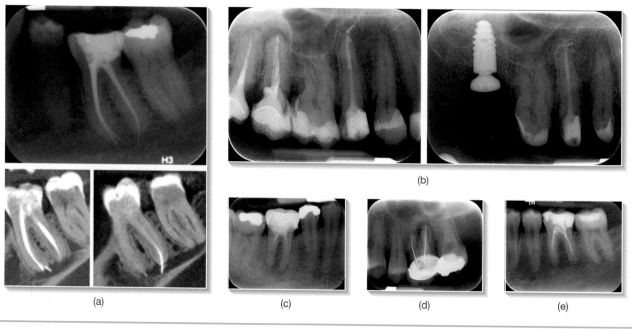

(a)   (b)   (c)   (d)   (e)

Endodontology at a Glance. First Edition. Alix Davies, Federico Foschi and Shanon Patel. © 2019 John Wiley & Sons, Ltd. Published 2019 by John Wiley & Sons, Ltd.
Companion website: www.wiley.com/go/davies/endodontology

Endodontics is the area of dentistry receiving the highest number of claims for compensation. This could be minimised by following established guidelines and protocols for procedures. The dentist must also ensure he/she maintains contemporaneous and accurate records, documenting all conversations, advice and treatment provided. Complaints and claims are most commonly related to the following areas.

Misdiagnosis of the cause of the pain

It can be difficult to identify the cause of the patient's pain, especially in those with irreversible pulpitis. It is therefore possible to provide root canal treatment on the wrong tooth. This risk can be minimised by ensuring a full history and assessment are completed, including all the relevant special tests, (see Chapters 4–7). Periapical radiographs must be of a high standard with findings correctly documented. If the history, examination and special tests do not clearly identify the cause of the pain, treatment should be delayed until the pain localises. If there is still uncertainty, a referral should be made to a specialist.

Recent restorative work causing pulpitis

Teeth that have had fillings or indirect restorations placed can develop pulpitis and consequently require endodontic intervention. This unexpected pain, additional cost and damage to their new restoration can cause considerable displeasure to the patient, especially if they had not been prewarned. Therefore, prior to proceeding with large fillings or indirect restorations, the patient should be advised of the risk that root canal treatment may be required in the future.

Lack of information available regarding options for management of the tooth

It is important that a patient is provided with all the suitable options for management: root canal treatment or retreatment, root end surgery, or extraction and replacement with an implant, bridge or denture. The advantages, disadvantages and approximate financial and biological costs of each suitable procedure should be discussed in order that the patient can make an informed decision about their treatment.

Failure to advise or offer referral to a more experienced practitioner

Root canal treatment is a difficult procedure to perform. Cases vary in complexity with poor access, sclerosis, severe curvature and retreatment cases presenting the greatest challenges. If dentists feel that a case is beyond their scope of expertise, they should advise the patient that they have the option to be referred to a specialist.

Complications during treatment

Complications occur, even when treatments are performed by experienced practitioners. Patients must be preoperatively warned of the likely risks of complications and, should one occur, the patient should be informed at an appropriate time during that treatment session. Rubber dam must always be used when performing endodontic procedures to prevent patient inhalation of instruments, ingestion of solutions such as sodium hypochlorite and to prevent further bacterial contamination of the root canals. Complaints arise because of the following complications:

- **Fractured instruments** Instruments fracture because of flexural or torsional fatigue (see Chapter 14). This risk can be minimised by adjusting the access cavity to improve straight line access to the canals and using files in a sequential manner with irrigation and lubrication. If rotary instruments are used, a suitable endodontic motor with a reducing handpiece must be used, and the appropriate torque and speed selected. The presence of a fractured instrument does not automatically result in failure of the procedure (Figure 36.1) but appropriate follow-up is necessary. Informing the patient of the occurrence of a file separation is mandatory for the clinician.
- **Perforation** Perforations can occur at various locations during root canal treatment (Figure 36.2). The risk of perforation is decreased by removing all the restorations to improve visibility and improving straight line access to the canals. Management of perforations is described in Chapter 17; a specialist referral is advised.
- **Hypochlorite accident** Sodium hypochlorite must be used with care to prevent splashes on the patient's clothes, skin or eyes. If it is extruded through the apical foramen, the patient can develop intense pain, swelling and bleeding. It can also cause sinus or inferior dental nerve damage. Although hypochlorite accidents are rare, an occurrence can be so severe that patients should be prewarned of this possibility. Methods of reducing and managing this complication are described in Chapter 21.
- **Inadequate obturation of the root canal system** A short or poorly condensed root filling often reflects poor preparation and disinfection of the root canal system. These cases are associated with an increased risk of failure. Overfilling of the canal is also associated with complications (Figure 36.3a) and lower success rates. However, if the canal is adequately disinfected and sealed, prognosis can still be good (Figure 36.3b). The use of an apex locator and a working length or cone fit radiograph are required to confirm the correct length prior to obturation. Materials such as silver points and resins (36.3c, d and e) fall short of the required standards and should no longer be used. Any outcome falling short of the expected standard level and its implications should be discussed with the patient.

Fracture of the tooth after treatment

Root treated teeth are at an increased risk of fracture (see Chapter 26). Patients should therefore be advised preoperatively that, once an adequate root filling has been placed and symptoms have resolved, a cuspal coverage restoration is necessary. An orthodontic band or a direct cuspal coverage restoration can be placed in the interim period. The occlusion should be adjusted to minimise the force placed on the tooth and the patient must be advised to exercise care when biting. Similar care should be paid between appointments for multi-stage root canal treatment.

Failure of the root canal treatment

Patients should be preoperatively advised that root canal treatment does not have a 100% success rate. If success rates are quoted, they should reflect the practitioner's own experience as the success rate of an inexperienced dentist is very different from that of a specialist. Patients should be advised that they will need to attend follow-up appointments to ensure healing occurs.

Index

Page numbers in *italics* refer to figures.
Page numbers in **bold** refer to tables.

Endodontology at a Glance. First Edition. Alix Davies, Federico Foschi and Shanon Patel. © 2019 John Wiley & Sons, Ltd. Published 2019 by John Wiley & Sons, Ltd.
Companion website: www.wiley.com/go/davies/endodontology

Notes

Notes

Notes

Notes